SIMPLY yoga

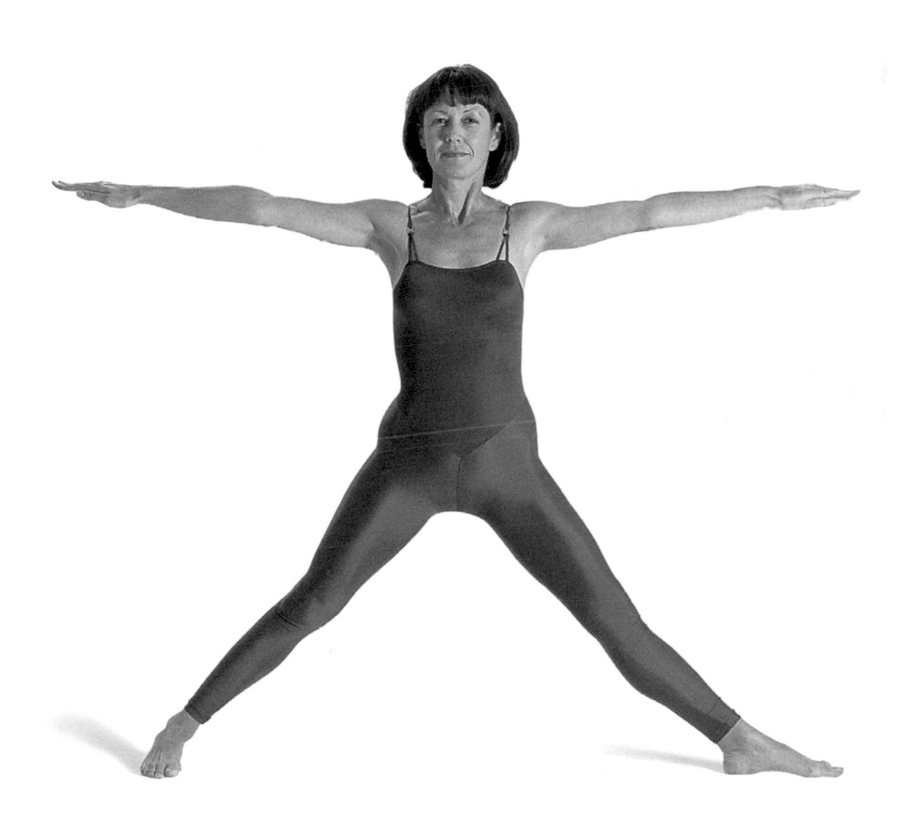

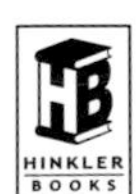

Box and book cover design: Hinkler Design Studio
Creative Director: Sam Grimmer
Photography: Peter Wakeman

First published in this format 2007
by Hinkler Books Pty Ltd
45–55 Fairchild Street
Heatherton Victoria 3202 Australia
www.hinklerbooks.com

HB01_SEP11_04

Printed and bound in China

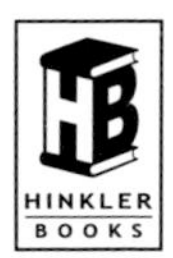

ISBN 978 1 7418 2042 3

Contents

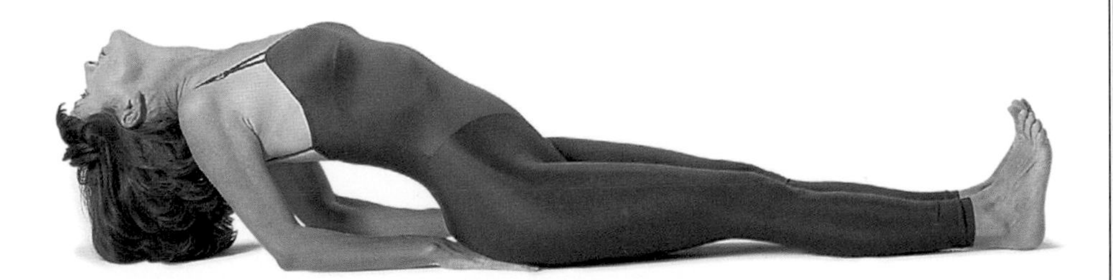

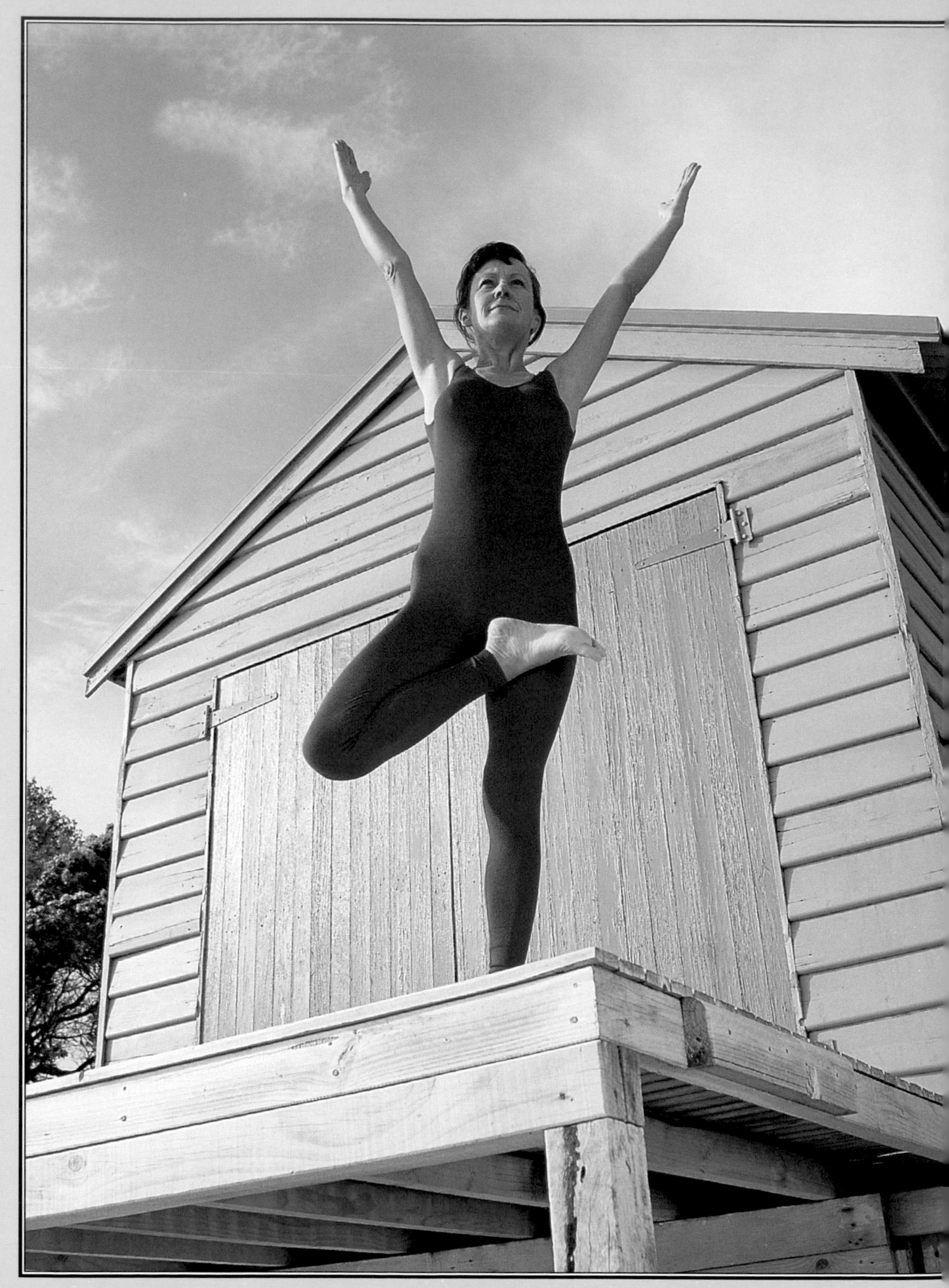

Introduction

This book is an easy guide to a balanced series of basic yoga postures. They are safe and effective for beginners and an excellent refresher course for the more experienced student.

The ancient science of yoga has been practised and passed on in the East for thousands of years, bringing health, happiness and peace of mind to those who have studied it. More recently, the benefits of yoga have been recognised and welcomed by the West and widely developed as a fitness regime. But the benefits are not merely physical. Yoga practitioners know that their quality of life improves on all levels – physical, emotional, mental and spiritual.

Here we are concerned with the physical aspects of yoga, but those of you who are able to practise the postures regularly will observe subtle and beautiful changes in other areas of your lives. Not only will your sense of physical wellbeing improve; feelings of stability, clarity and a greater capacity for concentration will emerge. Yoga can lift your capacity to succeed in all other areas of your life – work, study, sport, and in your relationships with others.

It is recommended that you begin with the opening Corpse Pose (Savasana) with its yoga breathing routine, and proceed to the following postures. The sequence has been designed so each posture will flow smoothly on to the next, through a variety of kneeling, sitting, standing and lying down practices, returning again to the final Savasana and a beautiful relaxation practice.

As individuals vary in strength and flexibility, so the practice of yoga will be unique to each individual. Your body will tell you where you are strong and which areas need more practice. Do not be disheartened if you cannot reach the full extension of a posture as shown. Daily gentle practice will encourage your body to release its tensions. On some days a particular posture may seem more difficult while another may seem easier. This is normal. Be gentle and accommodating with yourself. A daily routine will encourage your body to respond to the movements. Most of all, have fun. Enjoy reaching for your full potential.

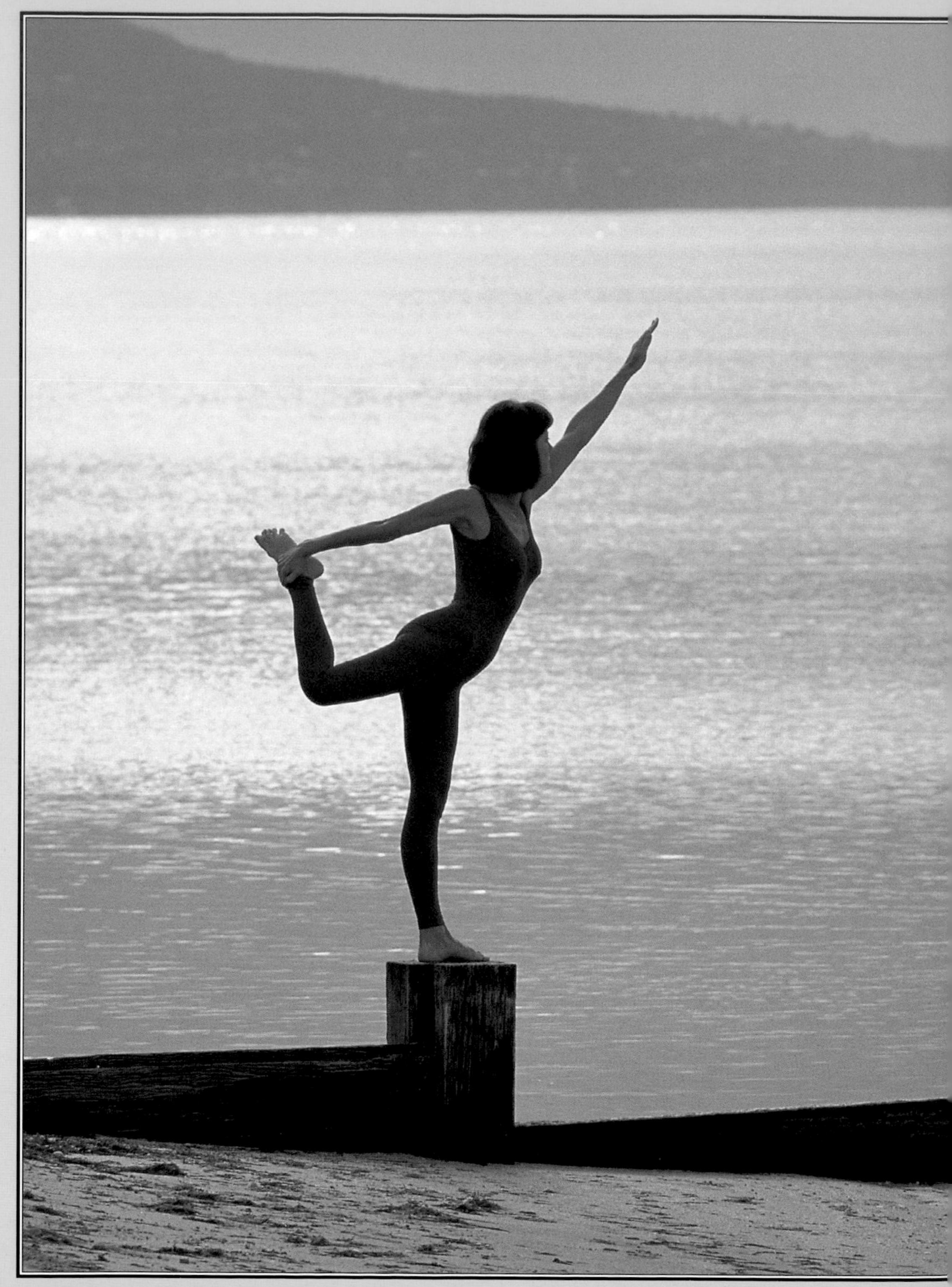

Practical Matters

It is important for you to follow the step-by-step directions and proceed at your own pace. As you do the postures, listen carefully to your body and recognise its warning signs. Rather than straining to achieve the required result, release your body gently into its own natural extensions. Do not try to push past pain. There is a difference between the feeling of stretching muscles and the pain associated with strain. If at any time you experience pain, slowly release out of the posture as you breathe out. Practised gently and regularly, the postures will increase your levels of fitness and flexibility.

A simple guide to the link between the breath and the body's movements during the postures: breathe in as the body stretches and expands; breathe out as the body contracts or folds forward. If there is no breathing instruction to follow, breathe normally.

Consult your health professional if you are in any doubt about your medical condition.

It is best to practise yoga when your stomach is empty. Before breakfast is ideal, or at least one hour before your evening meal.

Requirements

A good yoga mat provides a soft non-slip surface. A rug or carpet are also suitable surfaces on which to practice.

Folded blankets and a small cushion are helpful for easing strain in certain postures. It is recommended that you cover yourself with a blanket when resting, to avoid feeling cold.

Practise in bare feet and wear appropriate, unrestrictive clothing for ease of movement.

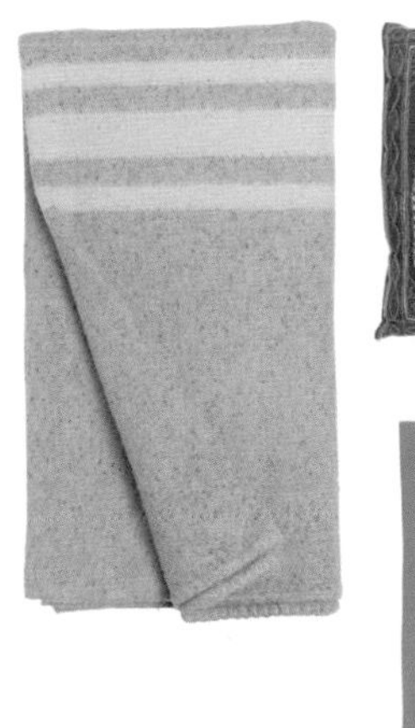

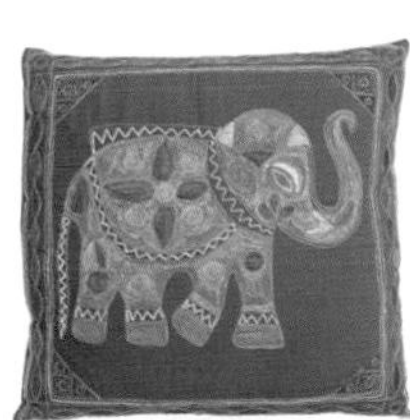

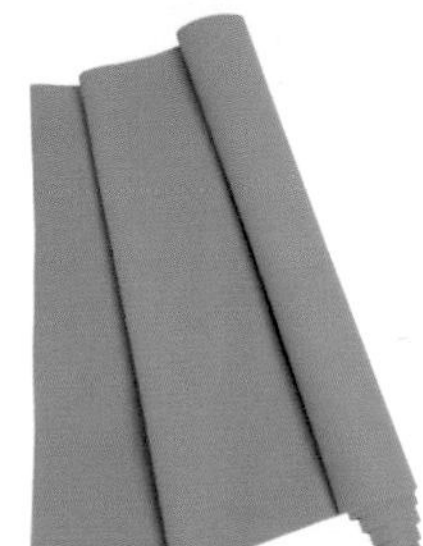

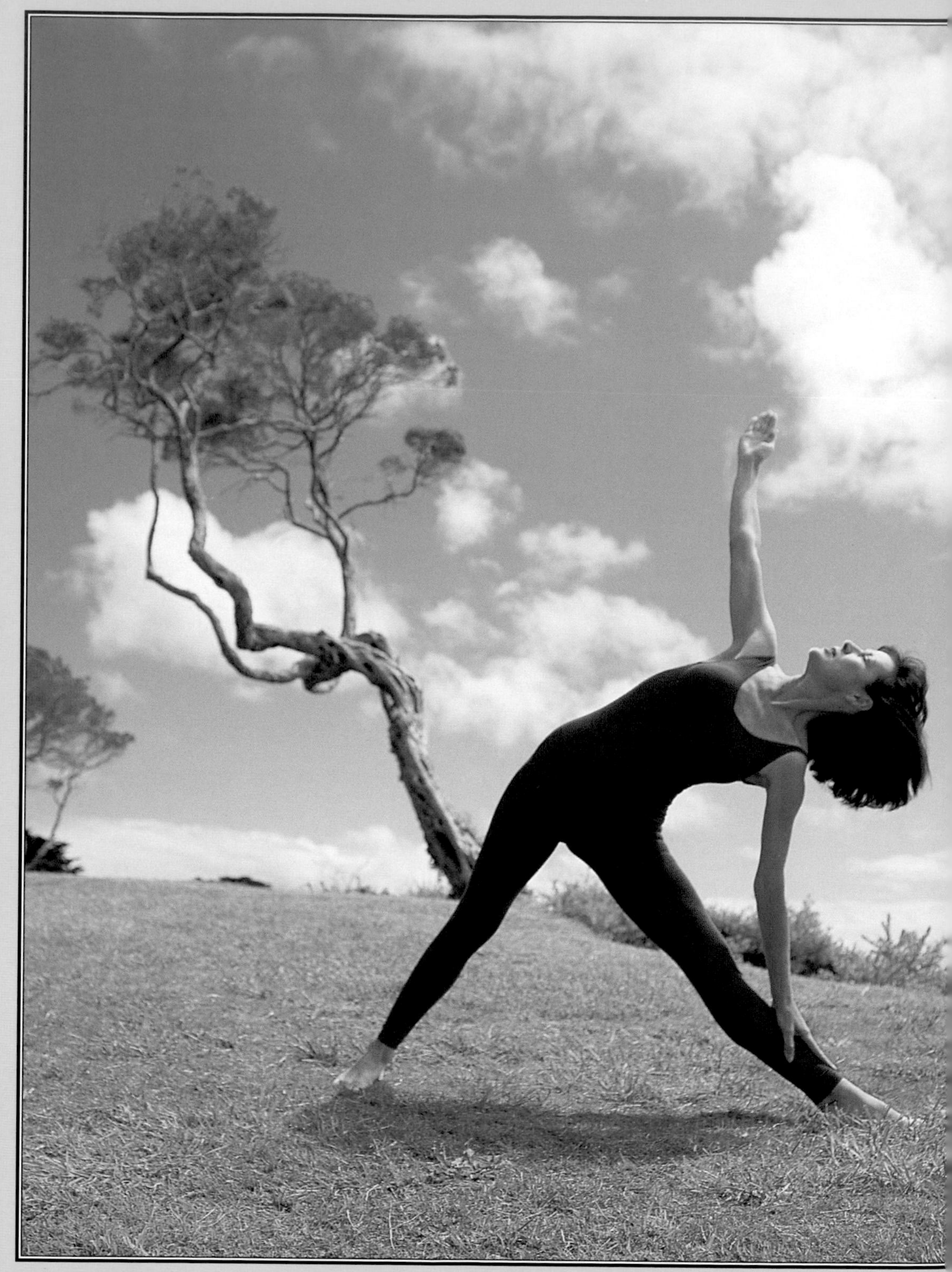

Yoga Breathing

Pranayama

Yoga breathing (Pranayama) is consciously observing the breath as we breathe in (inhale) and breathe out (exhale).

When the body is relaxed, the lungs are able to inhale and exhale more deeply. And the more deeply we exhale, the greater is our capacity to inhale fresh, clean air.

You will notice that yoga breathing involves breathing more deeply than your usual breathing. This deeper breathing brings more oxygen into your system. You may feel a little light-headed or dizzy when you begin. If you feel this happening at any time while doing the yoga postures (asanas), just take a moment to rest in the Child's Pose (Balasana).

The yoga breathing will change your usual pattern of breathing and will in turn change your state of mind. As your mind becomes clearer and more focused, your attention span will increase.

By beginning your yoga practice with a breathing sequence, you are increasing your mind's capacity to focus attention on the postures. As you follow the postures, continue to be aware of your breath.

There are many sequences of yoga breathing, but Lobular Breathing has been chosen as the ideal beginning to our simple posture sequence.

Lobular Breathing means breathing fully into the lobes of the lungs. We will breathe into the lower lobe (abdomen), the middle lobe (lower rib cage or diaphragm) and the upper lobe (top of the chest – just below the throat).

Yoga breathing is often practised in either the cross-legged pose (Sukasana) or the lotus pose (Padmasana). It can also be practised lying on the back in the relaxation pose (Savasana), and this is the way we will approach the breathing at the beginning of our practice.

Corpse Pose

Savasana

Before you begin your practice it is important to let go of the outside world, to focus your mind and body in preparation for the practices that follow.

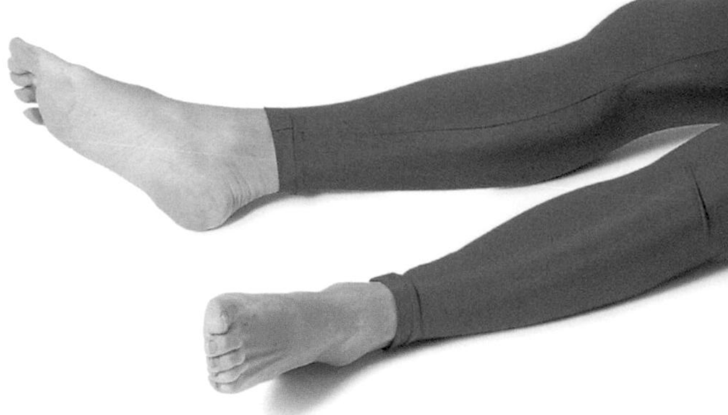

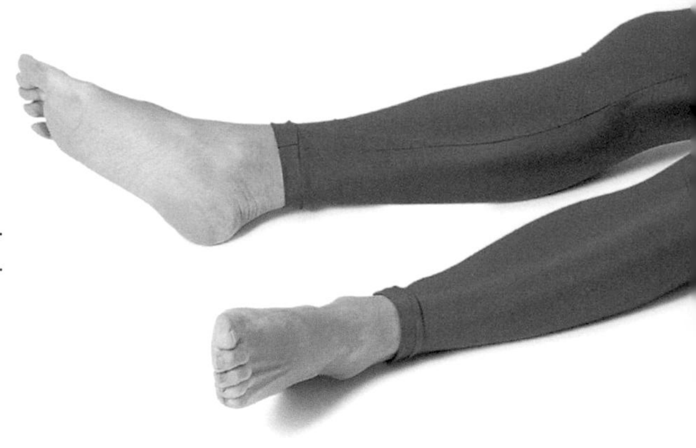

1 Lying on your back, relax your legs and allow your feet to fall outward. Relax your arms, turning the hands so the palms face upwards. Gently elongate your neck and allow the chin to tuck in slightly. Soften your face and close your eyes.

2 Breathe in and out through the nose, focusing your awareness on your breath.

3 Notice how you are feeling. Become aware of any tension, and as you breathe out, imagine the tension flowing out with the breath. As you breathe in, feel yourself filling up with positive, healing energy.

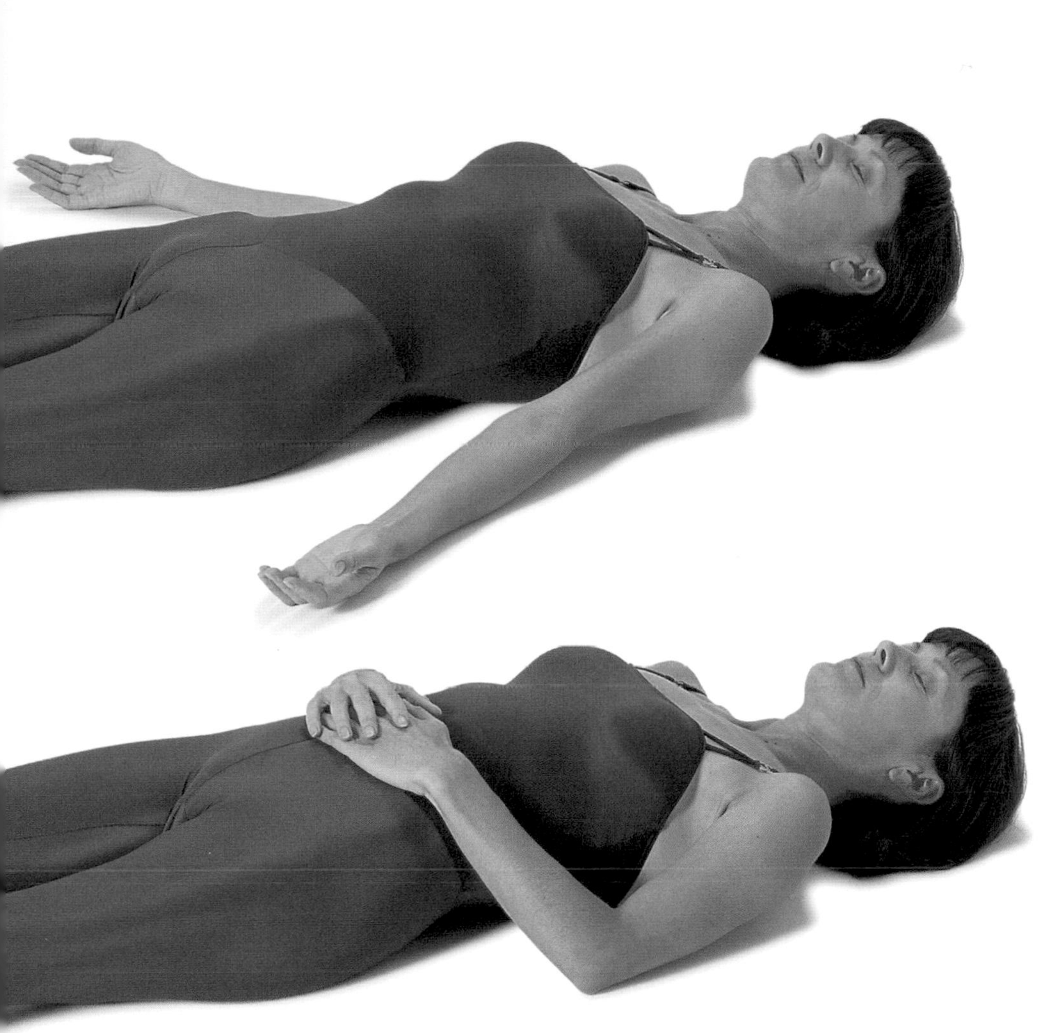

Breathing into the Abdomen

4 Gently place your hands one over the other, palms down, on your abdomen. Exhale slowly and completely. Then inhale, breathing into the abdomen, using the position of your hands to guide your breath. Allow the abdomen to rise and fill like a balloon. Hold your breath in momentarily, then slowly exhale. Hold without breath for a moment, then inhale again without rushing. Enjoy the feeling and the wonder of the breath. Breathe into the abdomen up to 5 times.

Corpse Pose

Savasana *(continued)*

Breathing into the Lower Rib Cage (Diaphragm)

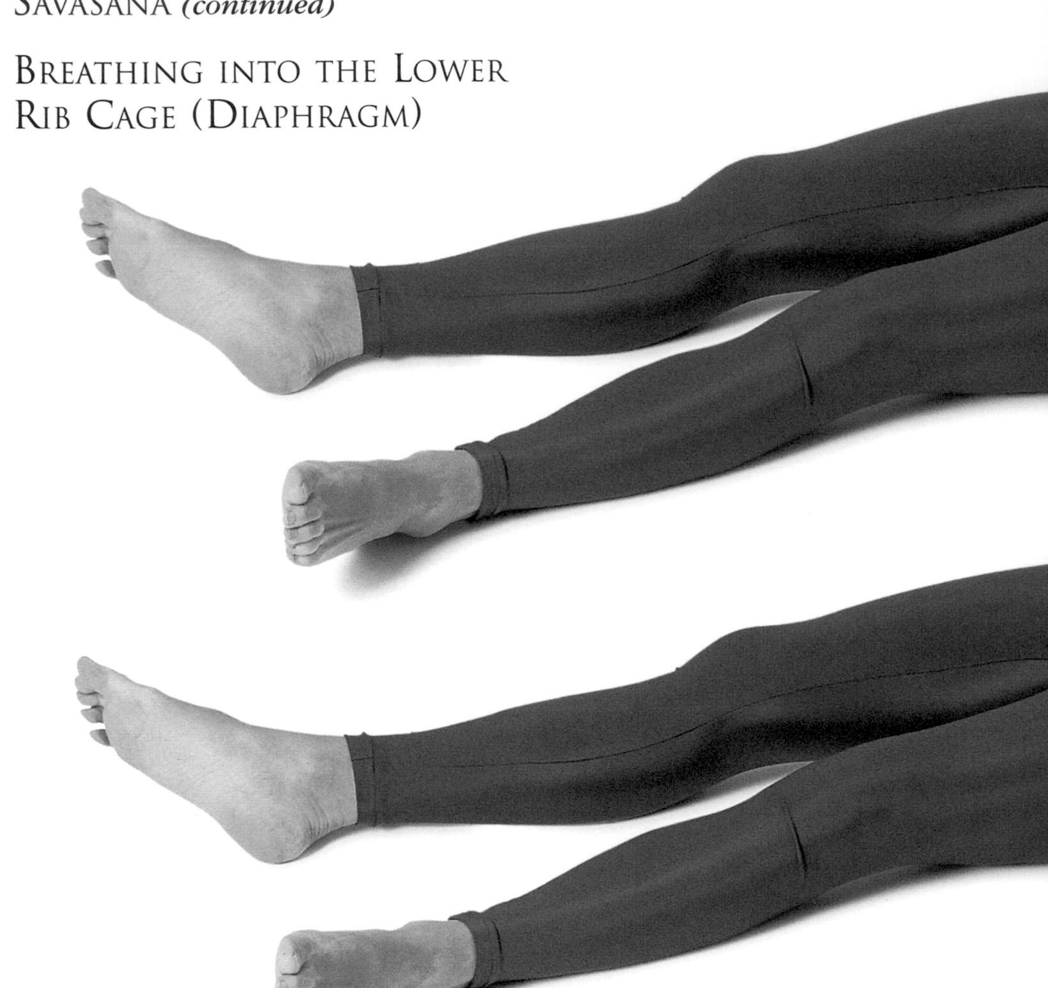

5 Place your hands at the base of the rib cage and exhale slowly and completely. As you inhale, breathe into the lower rib cage and feel the lower ribs expanding. Hold the breath in momentarily, then slowly exhale and feel the lower ribs contract again. Hold without breath for a moment before inhaling again. Breathe into the lower ribs up to 5 times.

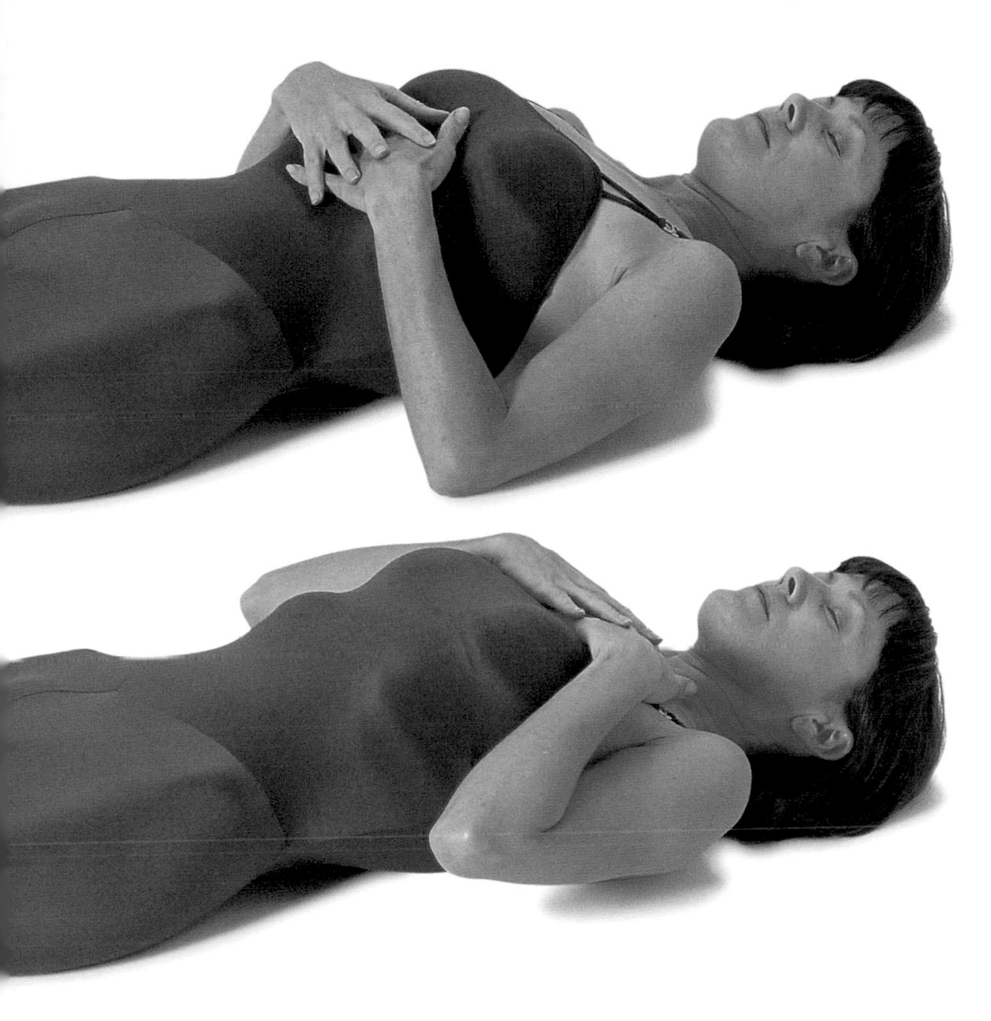

Breathing into the Upper Chest

6 Place the hands on the upper chest, below the throat. Exhale slowly and completely, then as you inhale, breathe slowly into the upper chest. You will feel a much deeper, fuller breath and you will feel expansion through the entire upper rib cage, front and back. Hold the breath for a moment before exhaling slowly and completely. Hold without breath for a moment, before inhaling again. Breathe into the upper chest up to 5 times.

Relax and take one or two normal breaths.

LIMBERING

Gentle exercises to prepare the body for the stronger postures that follow.

1 Lie on your back with your feet together and your arms by your sides. Slowly exhale.

2 Inhale as you slowly stretch your arms up over your head, lengthening through the whole body, stretching from the fingertips through to the toes.

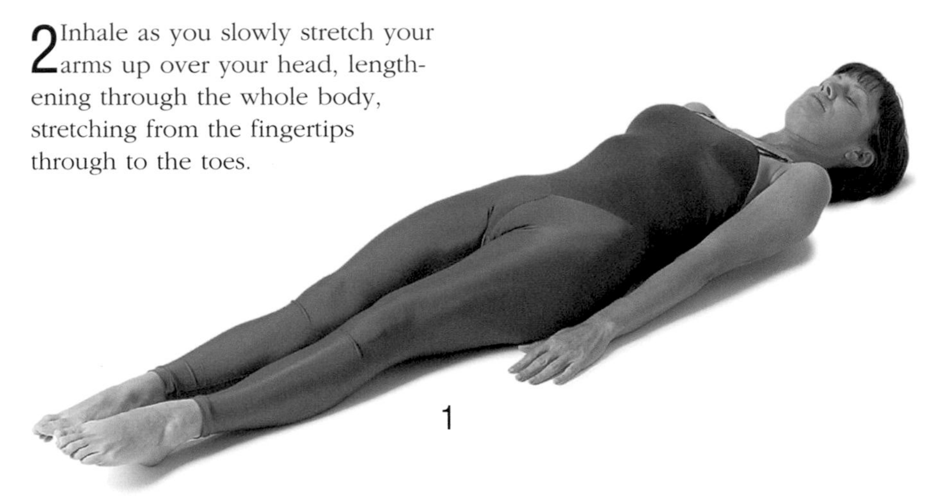

1

3 Exhale as you lift your arms up to the ceiling and down to your sides again.

4 Inhale as you draw your right knee towards your chest and place your hands around your knee. Exhale as you lift your head towards your knee, tucking your chin into your chest, and hold for a moment. Then release the knee and lower your head to the floor.

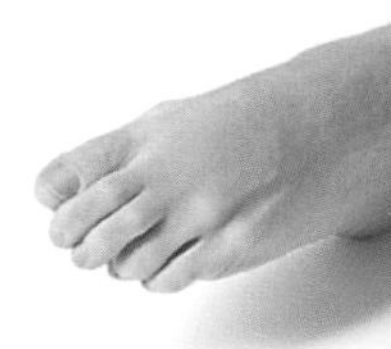

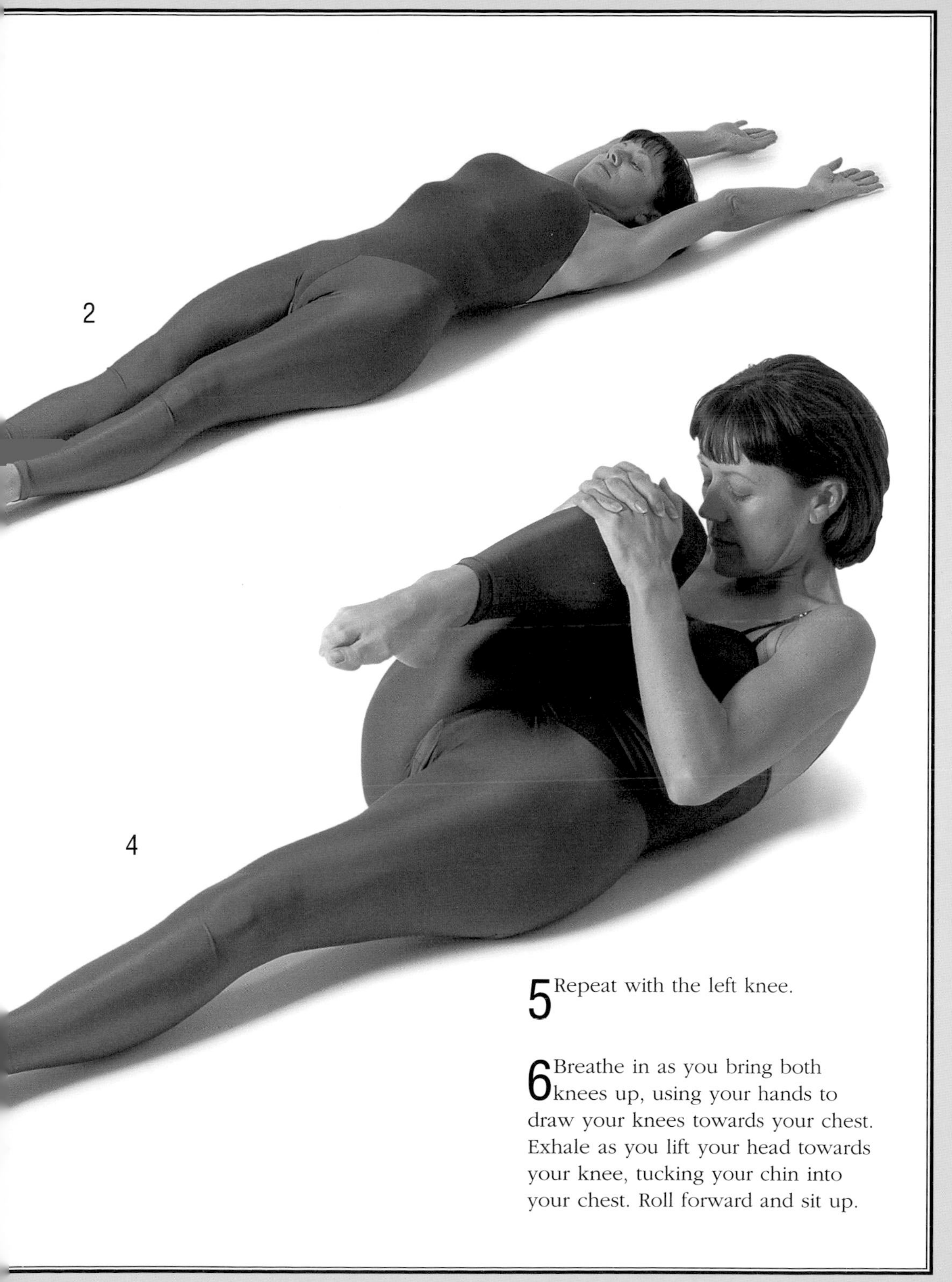

5 Repeat with the left knee.

6 Breathe in as you bring both knees up, using your hands to draw your knees towards your chest. Exhale as you lift your head towards your knee, tucking your chin into your chest. Roll forward and sit up.

Hero's Pose

Utthita Virasana

A kneeling stretch, this posture opens the shoulders and gives a full stretch to the spine.

1 Kneel on the floor, with knees together and the feet tucked under the buttocks. Rest the hands on the thighs. Tuck your chin in slightly. Open your chest, and feel your spine lengthening from the tail bone to the crown of the head.

2 Inhale and stretch your arms forward and continue the stretch until your arms are above your head.

3 Exhale as you bend forward and rest your forehead on the floor. Stretch your arms straight along the floor in front of you. Try to keep the buttocks down on the heels.

4 Hold this position for up to 5 breaths. Each time you breathe in draw the rib cage forward over the thighs. As you breathe out, lengthen the stretch from the fingertips to the tail bone.

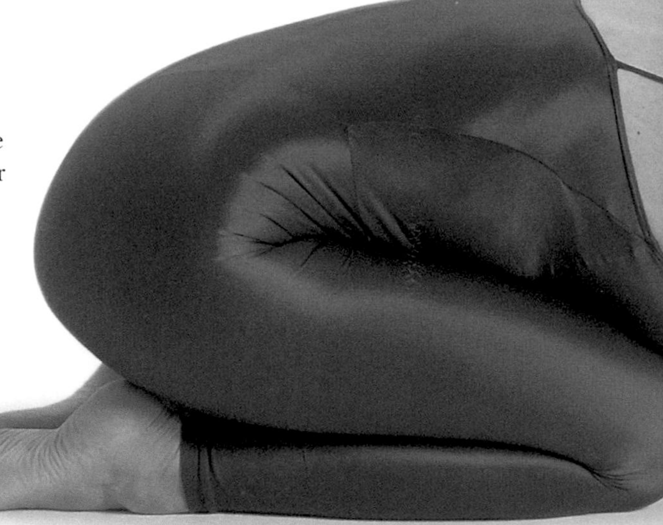

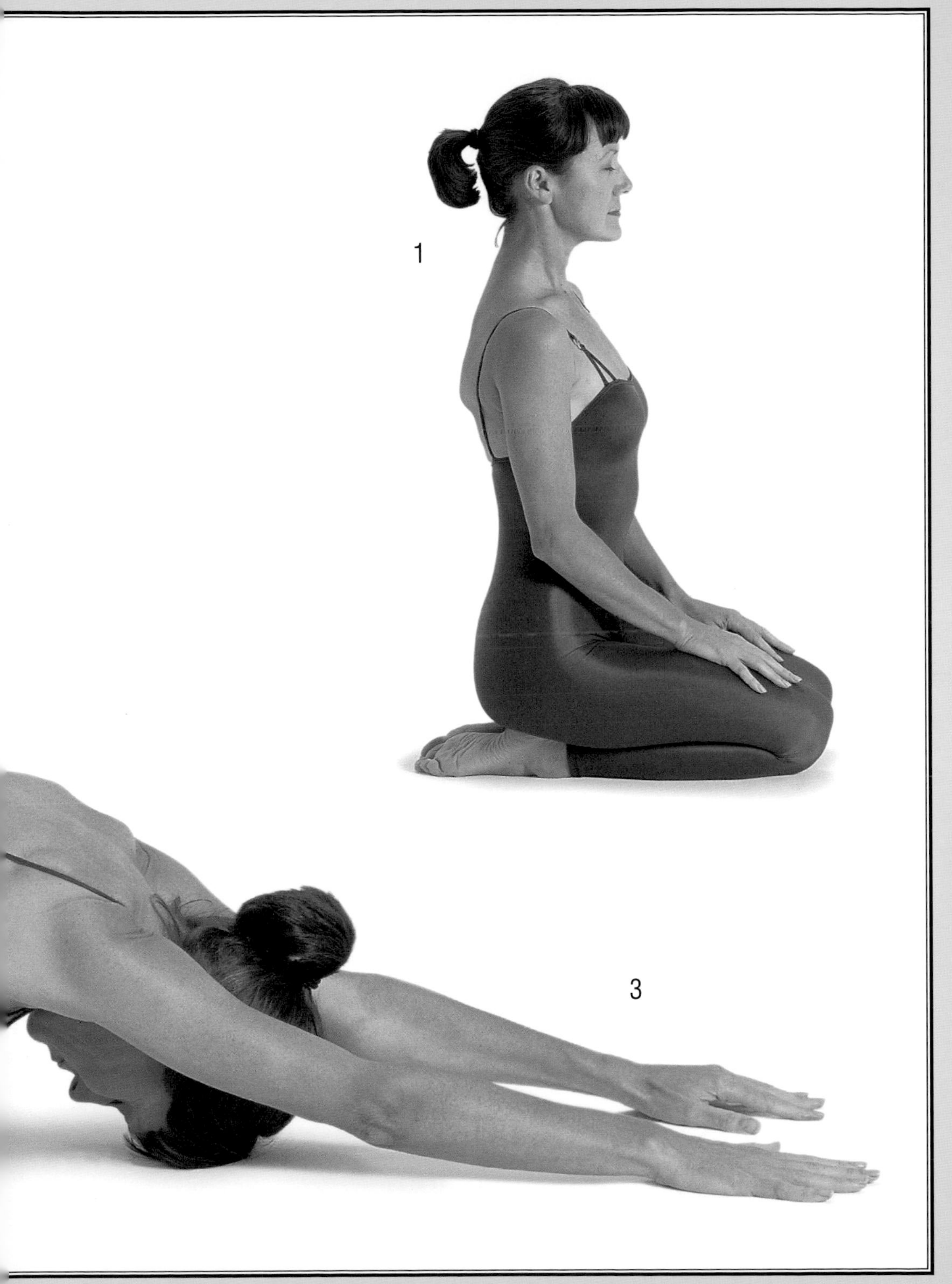
1
3

Cat Stretch

Giving a rhythmical spinal stretch, the cat stretch strengthens the shoulders, wrists, spine and hip joints.

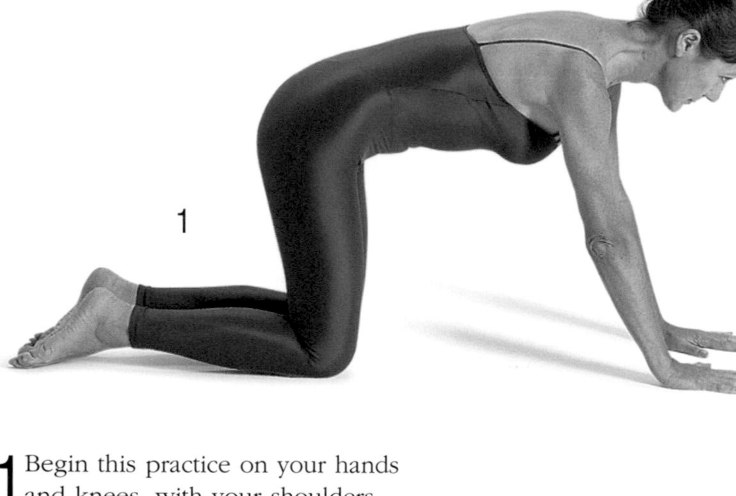

1 Begin this practice on your hands and knees, with your shoulders directly above your hands, and your hips directly above your knees.

2 Inhale as you roll your shoulders back and tilt your pelvis back and up. Tilt the chin and look up as the back concaves.

3 Exhale as you reverse the posture. Draw the abdomen in, squeezing all the breath out of it, as you arch your back. Tuck your chin into your chest and look down at your feet.

4 Continue concaving the back (inhaling) and arching the back (exhaling) gently and evenly, up to 5 times.

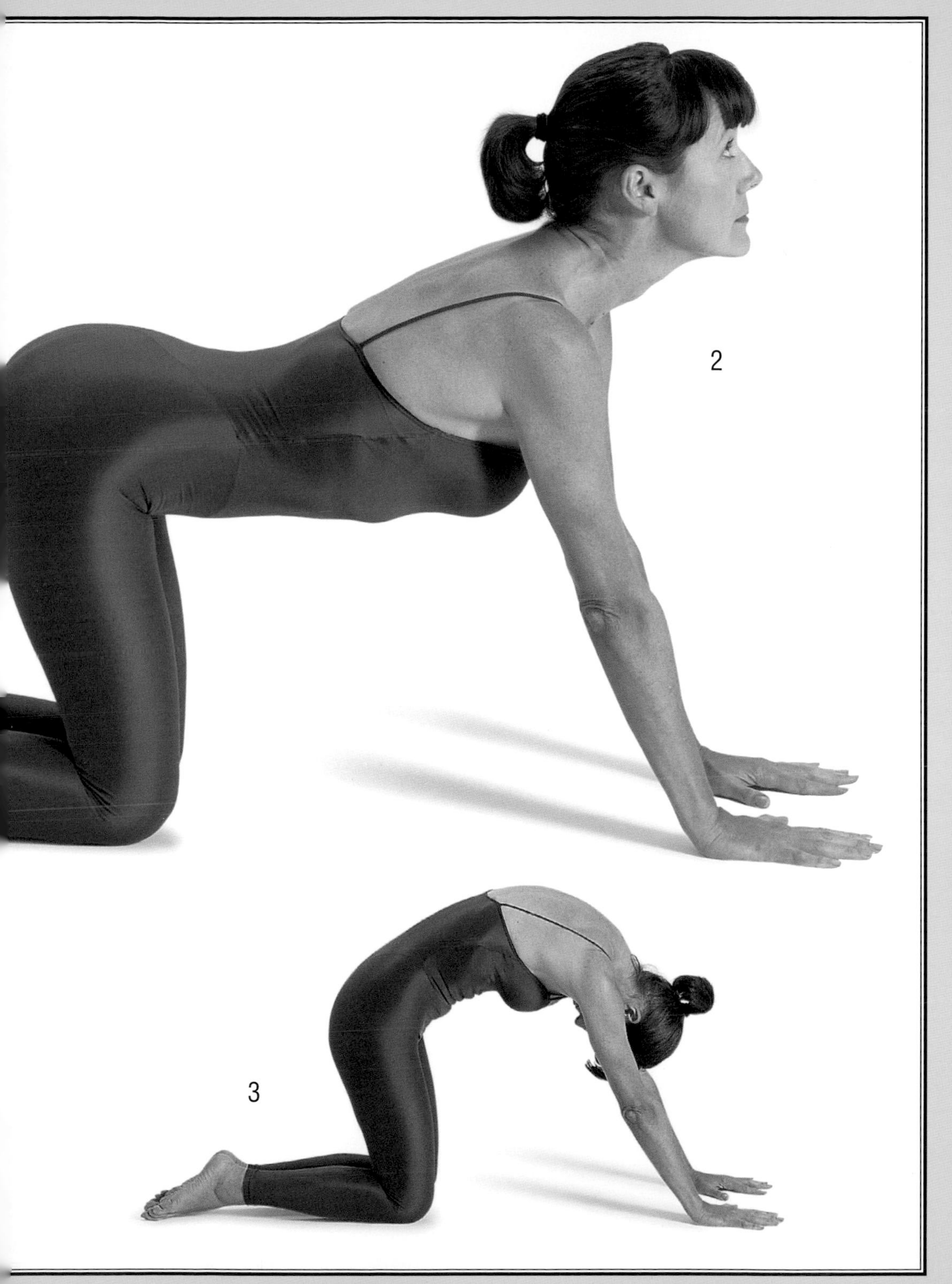
2
3

Child's Pose

Balasana

This is a beautiful resting pose. It relaxes the back, shoulders and the arms.

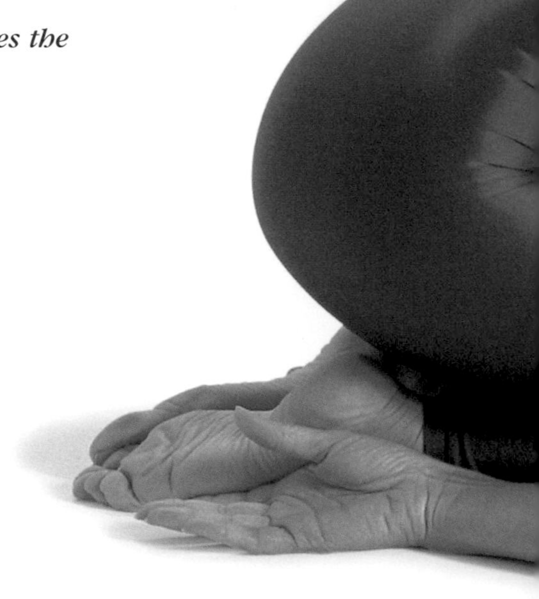

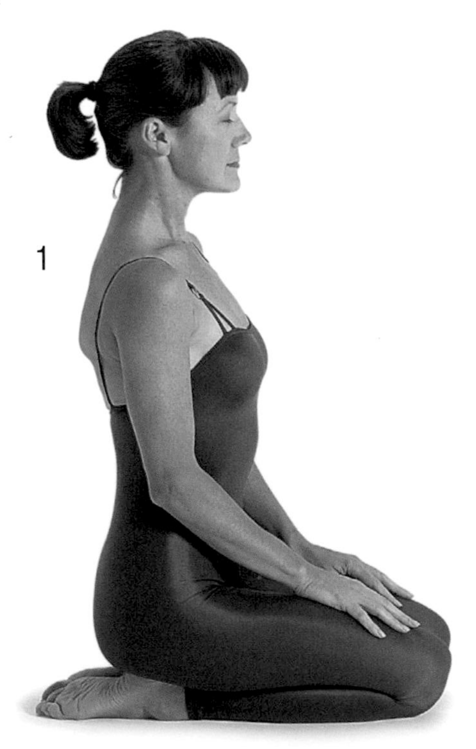

1

1 Kneel on the floor with your heels under your buttocks. Bend your torso forward so that your abdomen and chest are resting on your thighs. Tuck your chin under and allow your forehead to touch the floor. Bring your arms back so that they lie alongside the body, hands palm upward beside the feet. Soften the shoulders and the arms.

2 Bring your awareness to your breath. Breathe into any feelings of tightness. Let go of any tension with the exhaling breath. Rest in this pose before moving to the next posture.

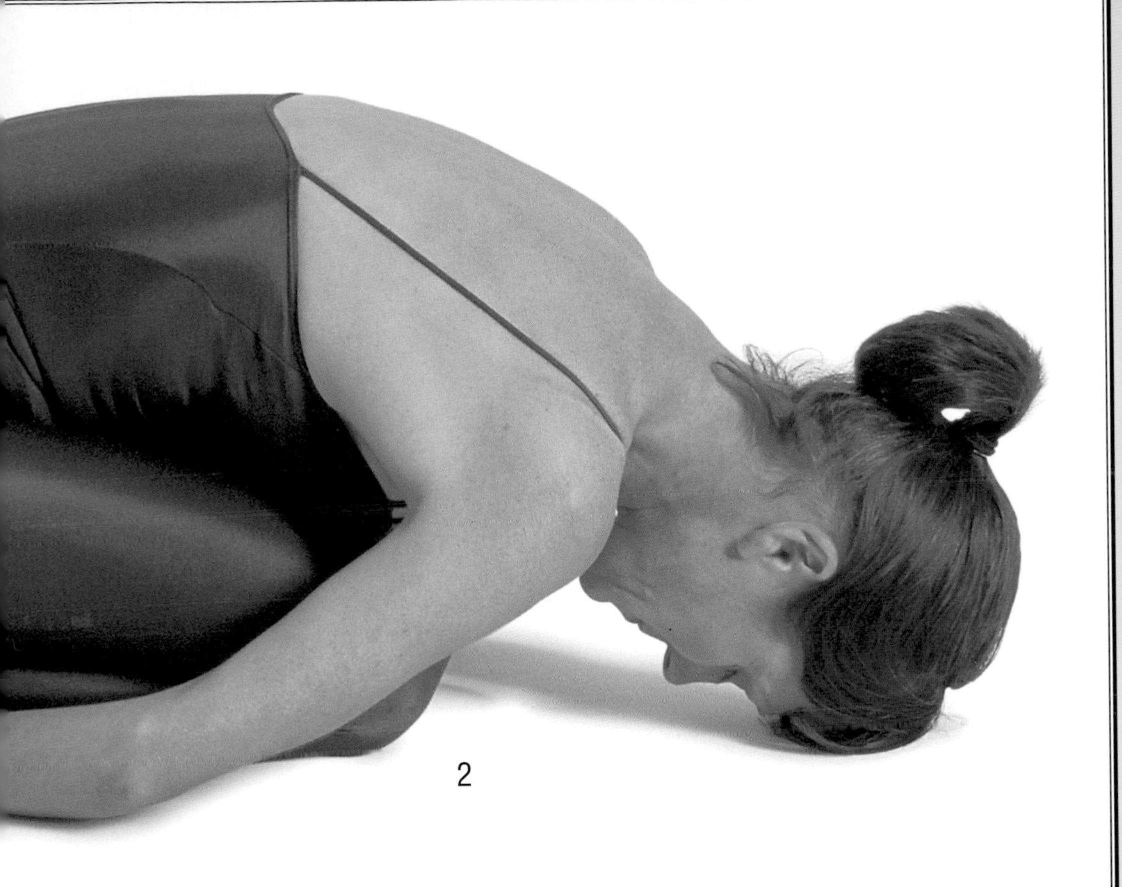

SOFTER

Kneel on the floor with your heels under your buttocks. Lean forward and rest your elbows on the floor a little further apart than your knees. Making fists of your hands, place one fist on top of the other. Rest your forehead on your fists. Follow step 2 on the previous page.

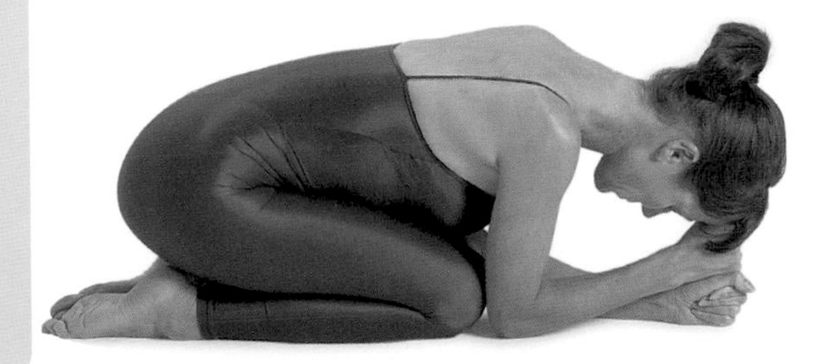

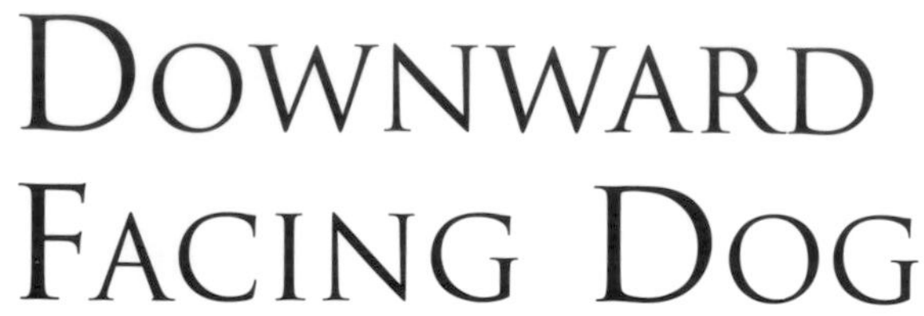

Downward Facing Dog

Adho Mukha Svanasana

This practice strengthens the shoulders, wrists and legs, and lengthens the hamstrings.

1 Kneel on all fours with your hands beneath your shoulders and your knees directly beneath your hips. Your feet should be at hip width apart. Spread your fingers wide apart.

2 Tuck your toes under. Inhale as you lift your body up, keeping your shoulders back and pushing backward into your hips. Keep your heels down as much as possible.

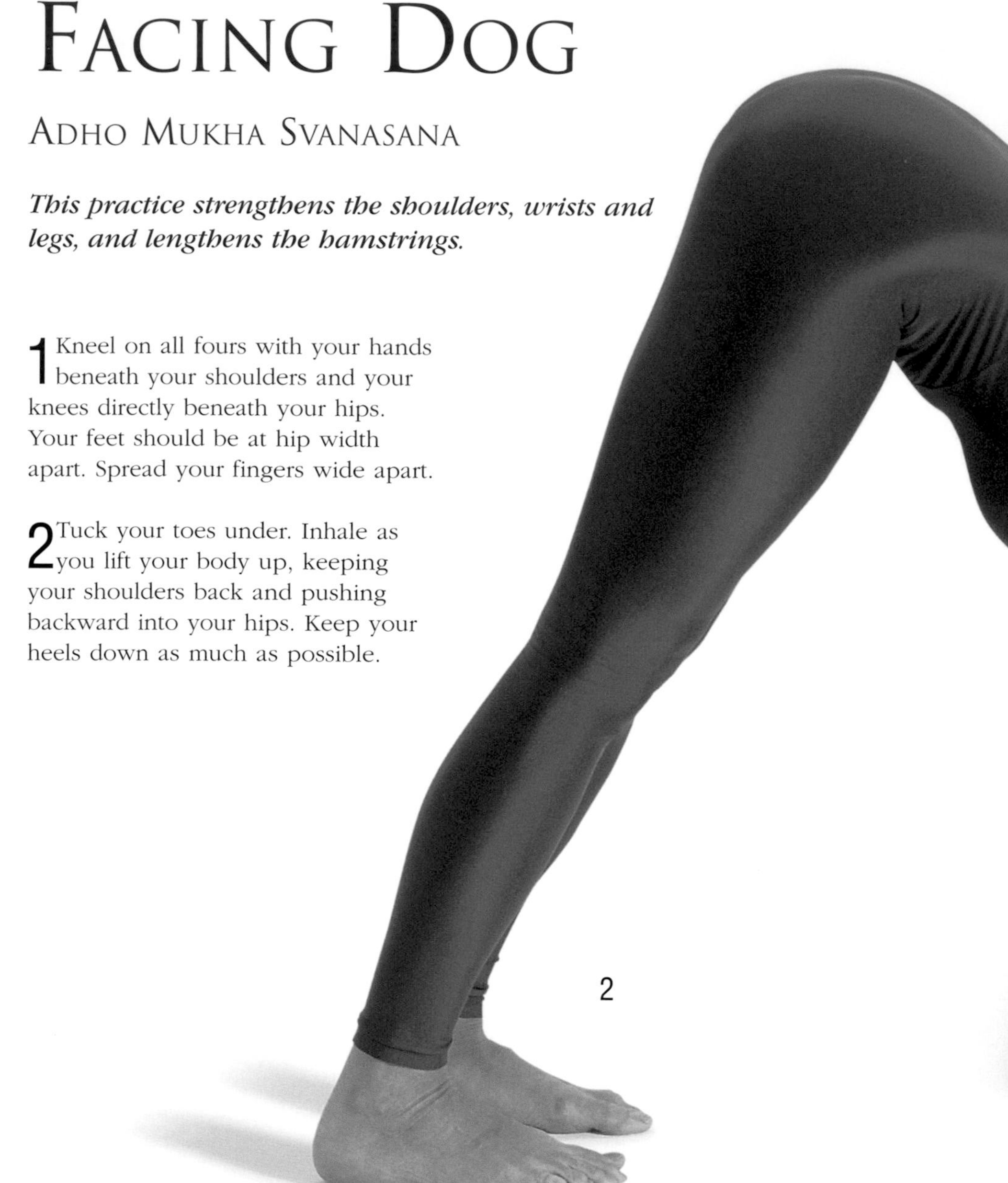

2

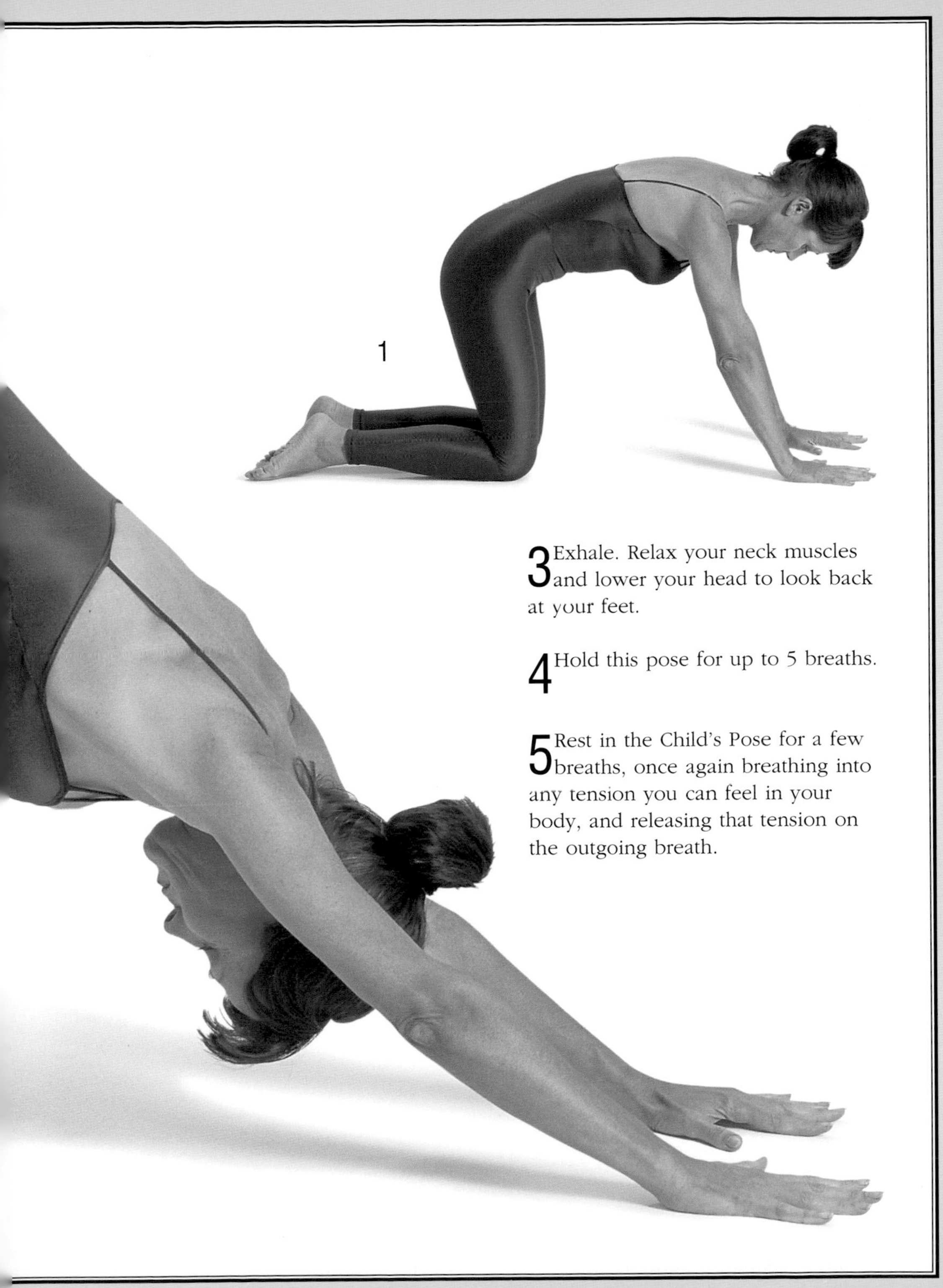

3 Exhale. Relax your neck muscles and lower your head to look back at your feet.

4 Hold this pose for up to 5 breaths.

5 Rest in the Child's Pose for a few breaths, once again breathing into any tension you can feel in your body, and releasing that tension on the outgoing breath.

The Cobra

Bhujangasana

This pose arches the back like the curve of a snake, toning and strengthening the vertebral muscles.

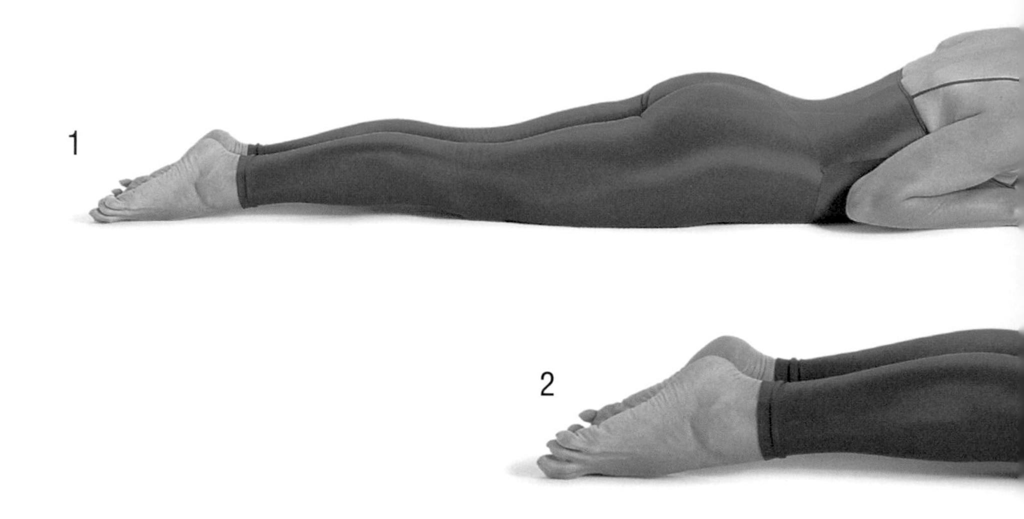

1 Lie on your front with your arms outstretched and your forehead touching the mat. Bring your arms back towards your body until your hands are directly beneath your shoulders. Keep your elbows tucked in beside the body.

2 As you inhale, lift your chin, your neck and then your chest, curving your spine up and back. Press down on the mat with your hands, gently increasing the arch in your back. Try to keep your feet together. Hold for 5 breaths.

3 Exhale as you release down in the reverse order – lowering your chest first, then your chin, then curve your head down until your forehead is once again on the mat.

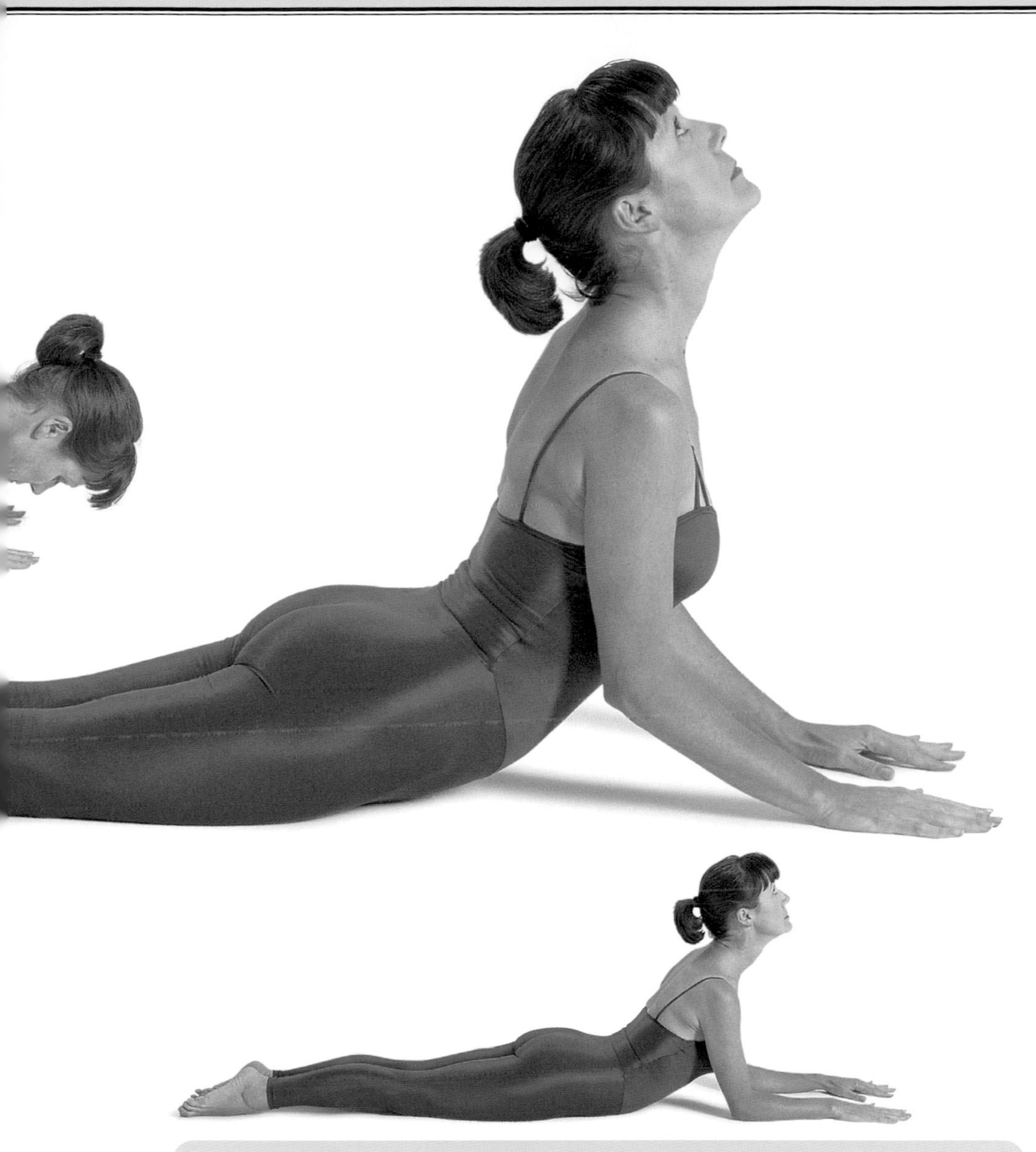

SOFTER

Lying in the outstretched position on your front, bring your arms back towards your body so that your elbows are directly under your shoulders. Your chest will lift a little to achieve this position. Inhale as you lift your head and chest up and roll your shoulders back. Straighten your arms and curve your spine up and back. Hold for up to 5 breaths. Exhale as you lower your torso in the reverse order – your chest first, then your chin, then your head.

STANDING FORWARD BEND

UTTANASANSA

This restful practice loosens the neck and shoulder muscles, extends the spine and strengthens the leg muscles.

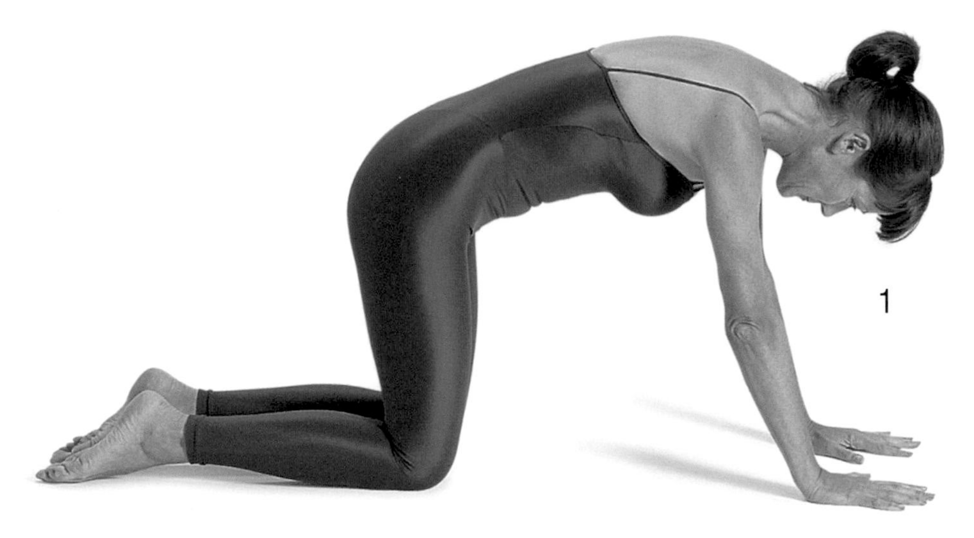

1

1 From the cobra pose, raise your body to the all-fours position and walk your knees in towards your hands.

2 Spread your fingers on the floor and tuck your toes under. Walk your hands back towards your knees.

3 Standing on your feet now, allow your head to continue to hang forward. Place your hands around your elbows.

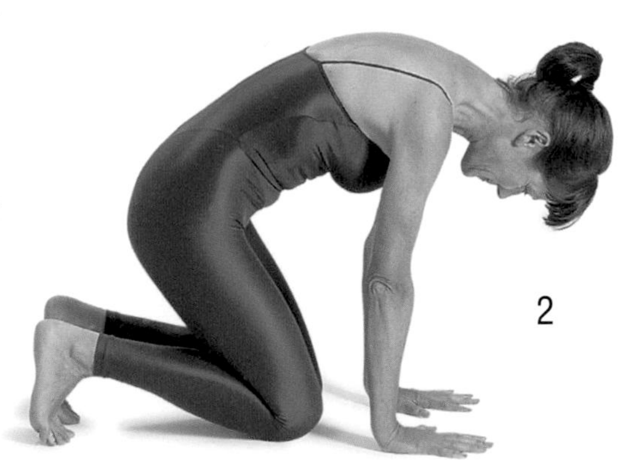

2

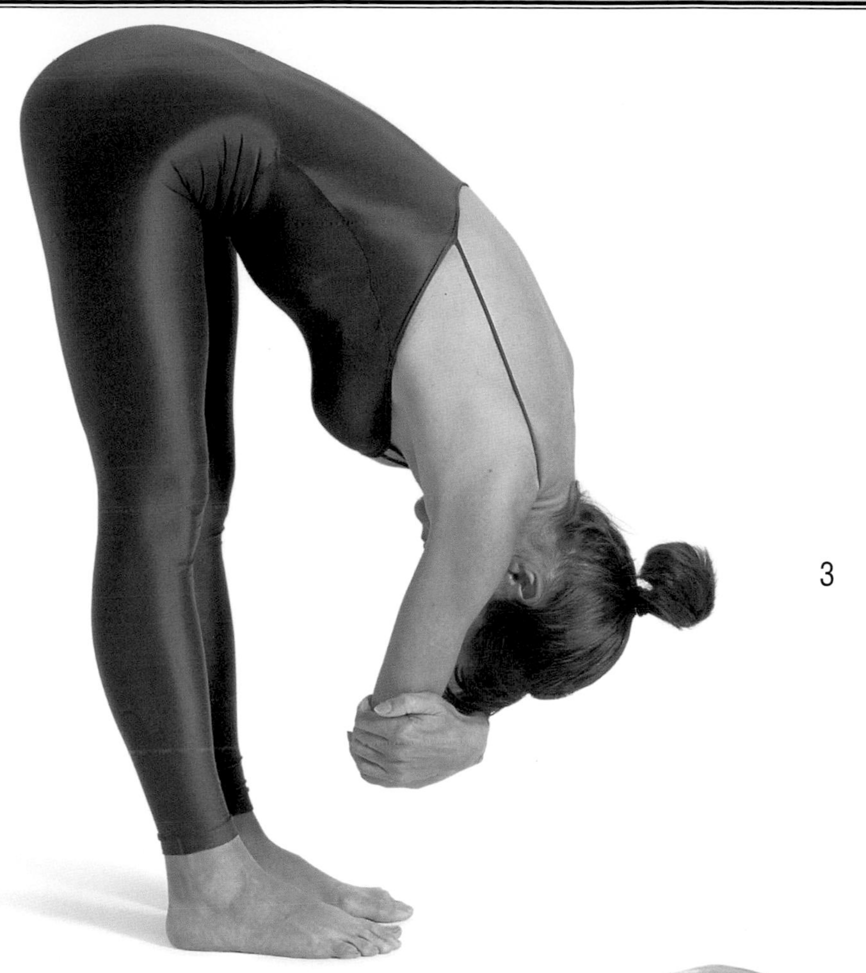

3

4 Each time you exhale, contract your abdomen and allow gravity to draw your torso down. Remember to keep your neck muscles soft. Hold this position for up to 5 breaths.

5 Exhale as you let your hands fall.

6 Inhale as you gently uncurl upwards, one vertebra at a time, until you reach the standing position. Allow your knees to bend if you feel any strain.

6

Shoulder Rotations

This practice releases any tightness in the neck and shoulders.

1 Stand with your feet at hip width apart and your arms hanging relaxed by your sides.

2 Inhale as you bring your shoulders up to your ears. Roll your shoulders firmly back. Squeeze them as close together as you can. Then exhale as you roll them downward and return to the starting position.

3 Inhale as you squeeze your shoulders together behind you. Bring them up to your ears, and exhale as you roll them forward and down.

4 Continue rotating your shoulders up to 5 times forwards and backwards.

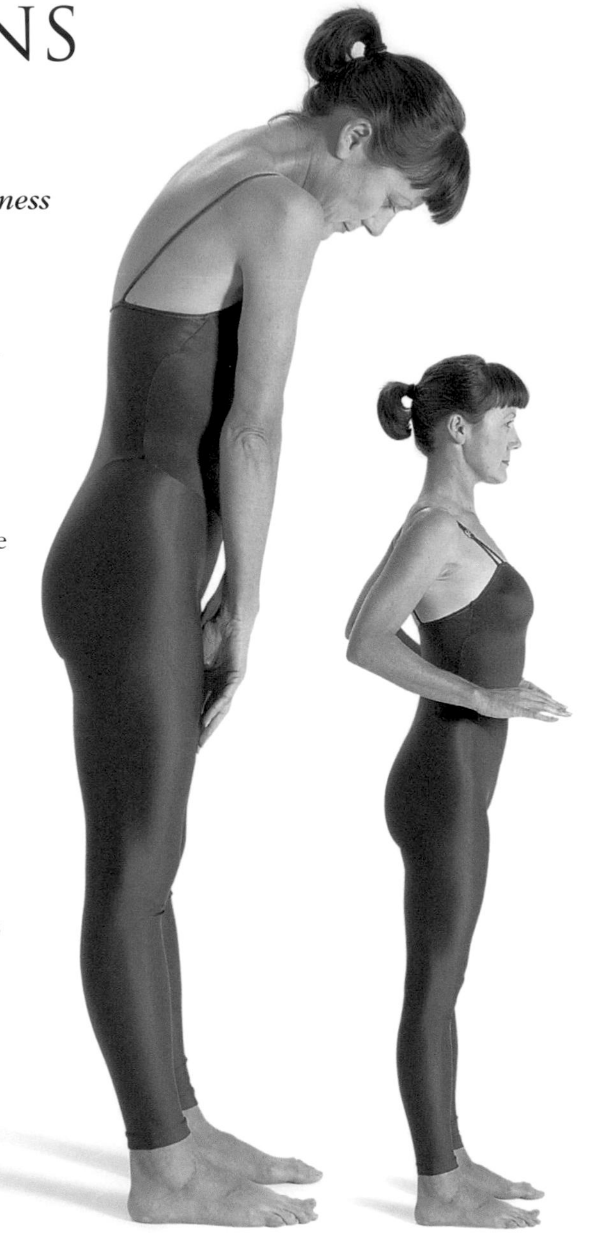

Mountain Pose

Tadasana

This simple pose encourages balance, good posture, elongation of the spine, and vertebral alignment.

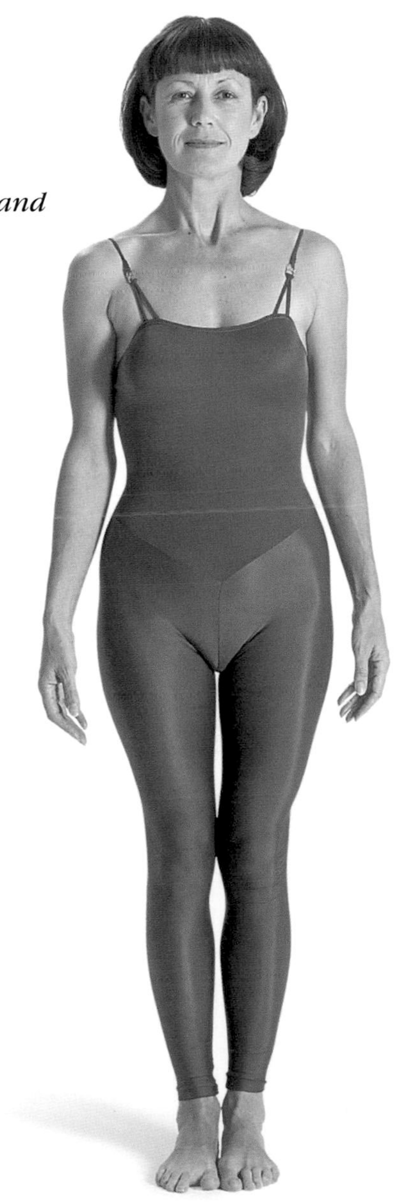

1 Stand with your feet together, your arms relaxed by your sides and your weight evenly balanced over the feet. Keep your chest open. Look straight ahead and soften your gaze.

2 Gently 'lift' the knee and thigh muscles, tuck your tail bone under and abdomen in. Feel your spine lengthen from the tail bone to the crown of your head. Allow the back of your head to lift slightly and tuck your chin in.

3 Remain steady but continue to 'lift' and stand tall. Hold for up to 5 breaths.

Chair Pose

Utkatasana

A standing posture that strengthens the shins, knees, thighs and hips.

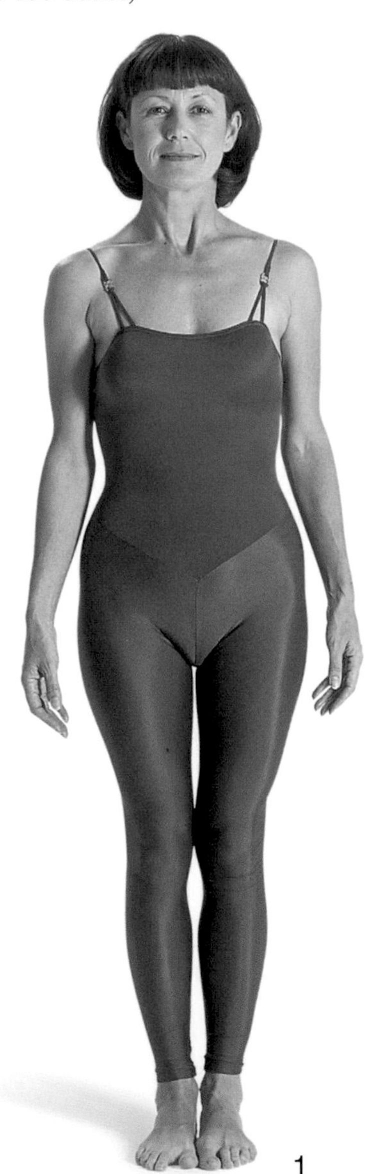

1 Stand with your feet together in the Mountain Pose, keeping your back tall and straight.

2 Lift your arms straight above your head. Your upper arms should be directly beside your ears. Tuck your chin in slightly. Place your hands in the prayer position with the thumbs locked.

3 Tucking your tailbone under, exhale as you squat as if to sit on a chair.

4 Hold for up to 5 breaths. On each outward breath, sink a little deeper while maintaining the upward stretch.

5 Inhale as you straighten your legs and return to the standing position.

SOFTER

As you exhale, sink into the sitting position, and as you inhale, straighten your legs to the standing position. Do this up to 5 times.

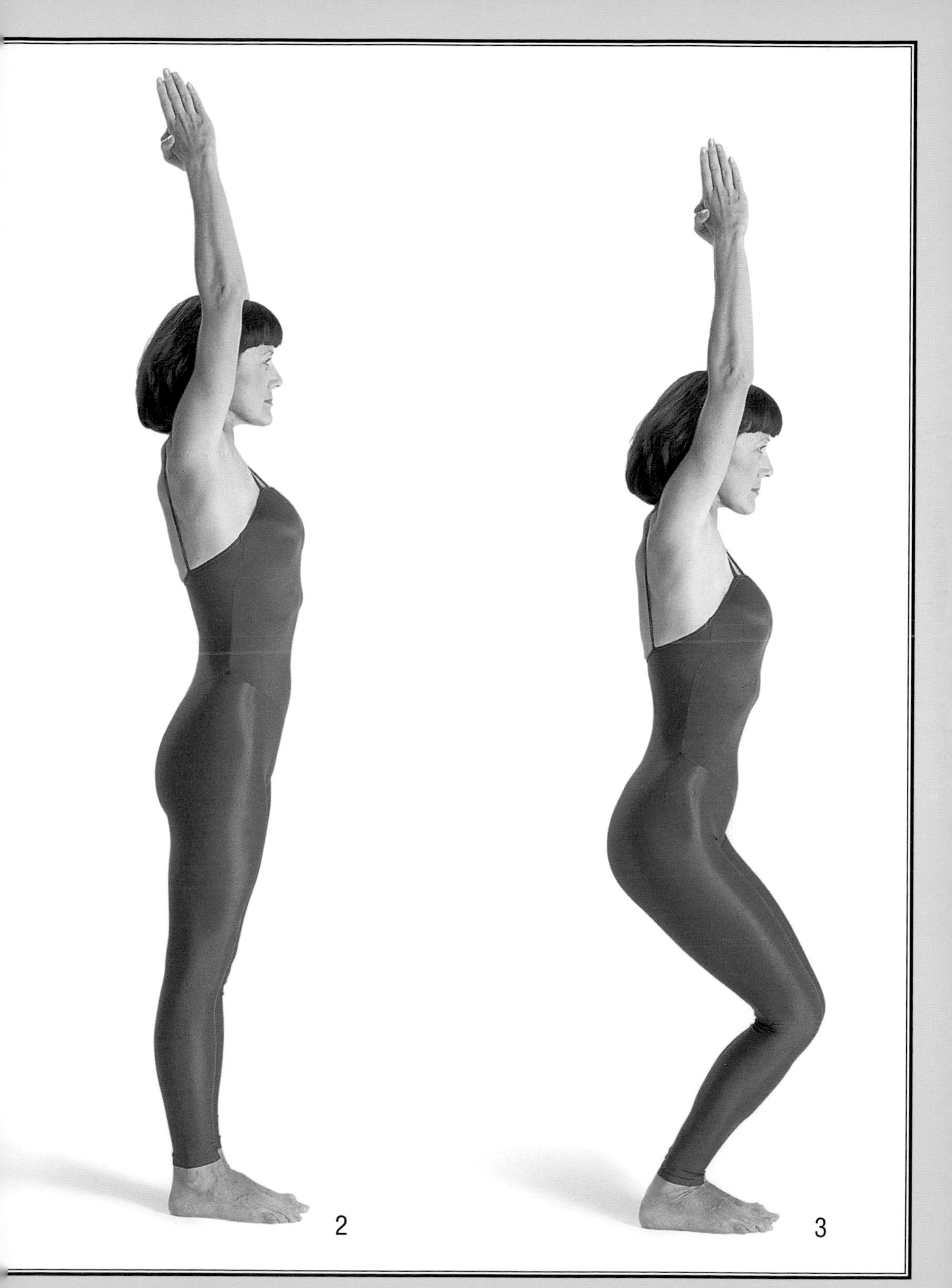
2
3

Triangle Pose

Trikonasana

This is a strong posture for opening and stretching the shoulders. It will also tone the back, the hips and the inner thighs.

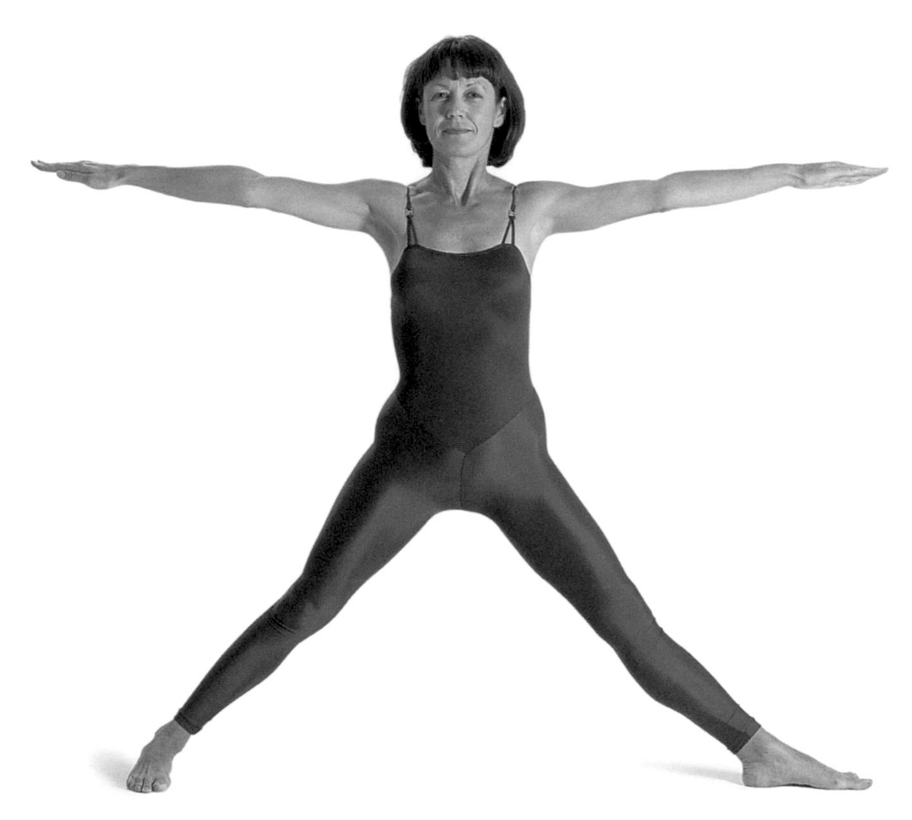

1 Stand with your feet a little more than 1 metre apart. Point your right foot straight ahead. Turn your left foot at right angles to it, to the left.

2 Inhale and stretch both arms out to the sides at shoulder level with the palms facing downward. Roll your shoulders back. Exhale.

3 Inhale, keeping your hips and shoulders facing forward. Exhale as you slide your left hand down your left leg. Your right shoulder should stay open in alignment with the left shoulder. Raise the right arm with the fingers straight as arrows as the left arm goes down. Take care not to tilt or twist the body while you raise the right arm. Gently 'lift' the thighs and the kneecaps. Look up at the raised hand if possible.

4 Hold for up to 5 breaths. Each time you inhale, lengthen the stretch upward. Each time you exhale, slide the left arm a little further down the leg.

SOFTER

Slide the left hand down only as far as the knee. The right arm is placed on the hip. If possible, the head should still turn and look up to the right, even if only managed for short periods. Repeat to the other side.

5 To release out of this posture, lower the raised arm, turn your head and look down at your ankle and allow your knee to bend. Gently return to the standing position,with your head and feet aligned to the front. Repeat to other side.

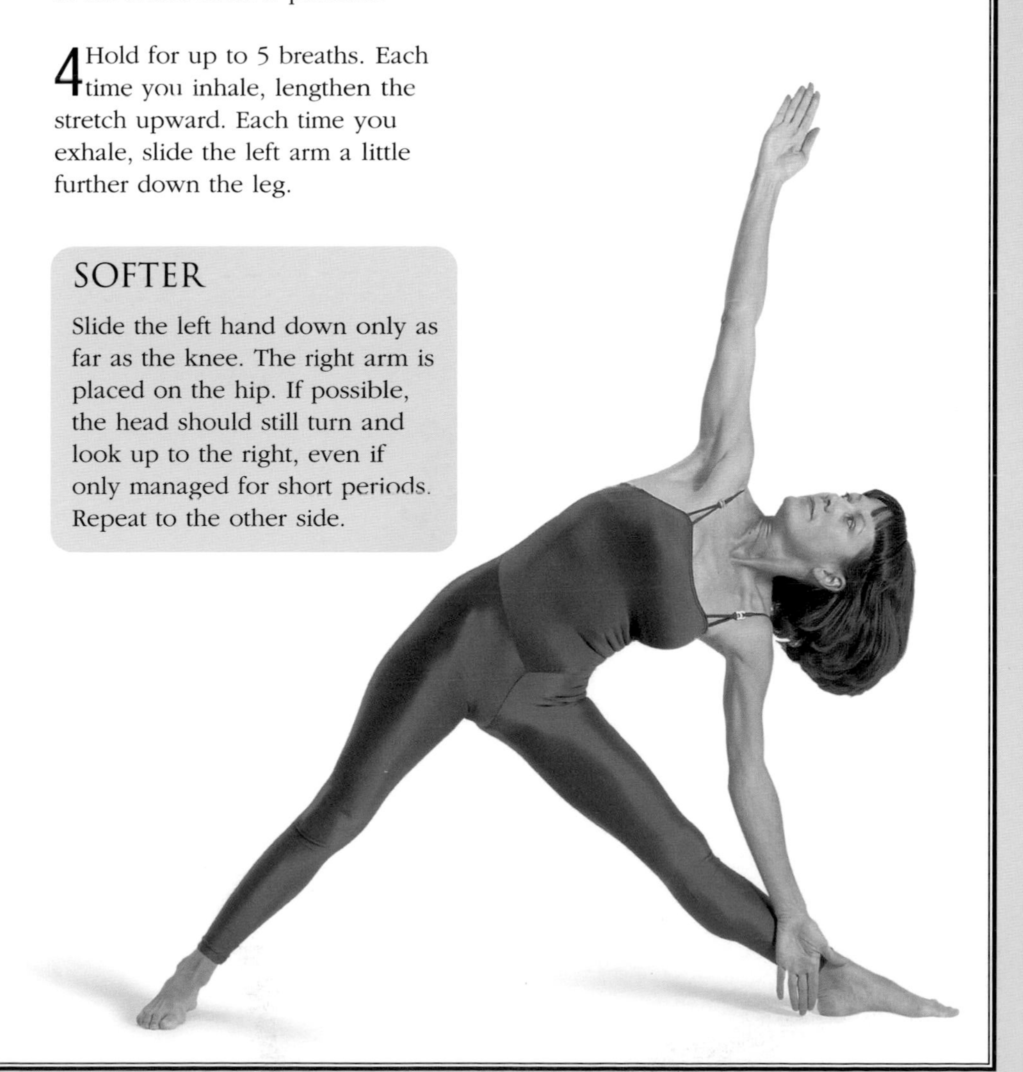

WARRIOR POSE

VIRABHADRASANA

This strengthening practice opens the hips and the shoulders, tones the arms, lower back, thighs and knees.

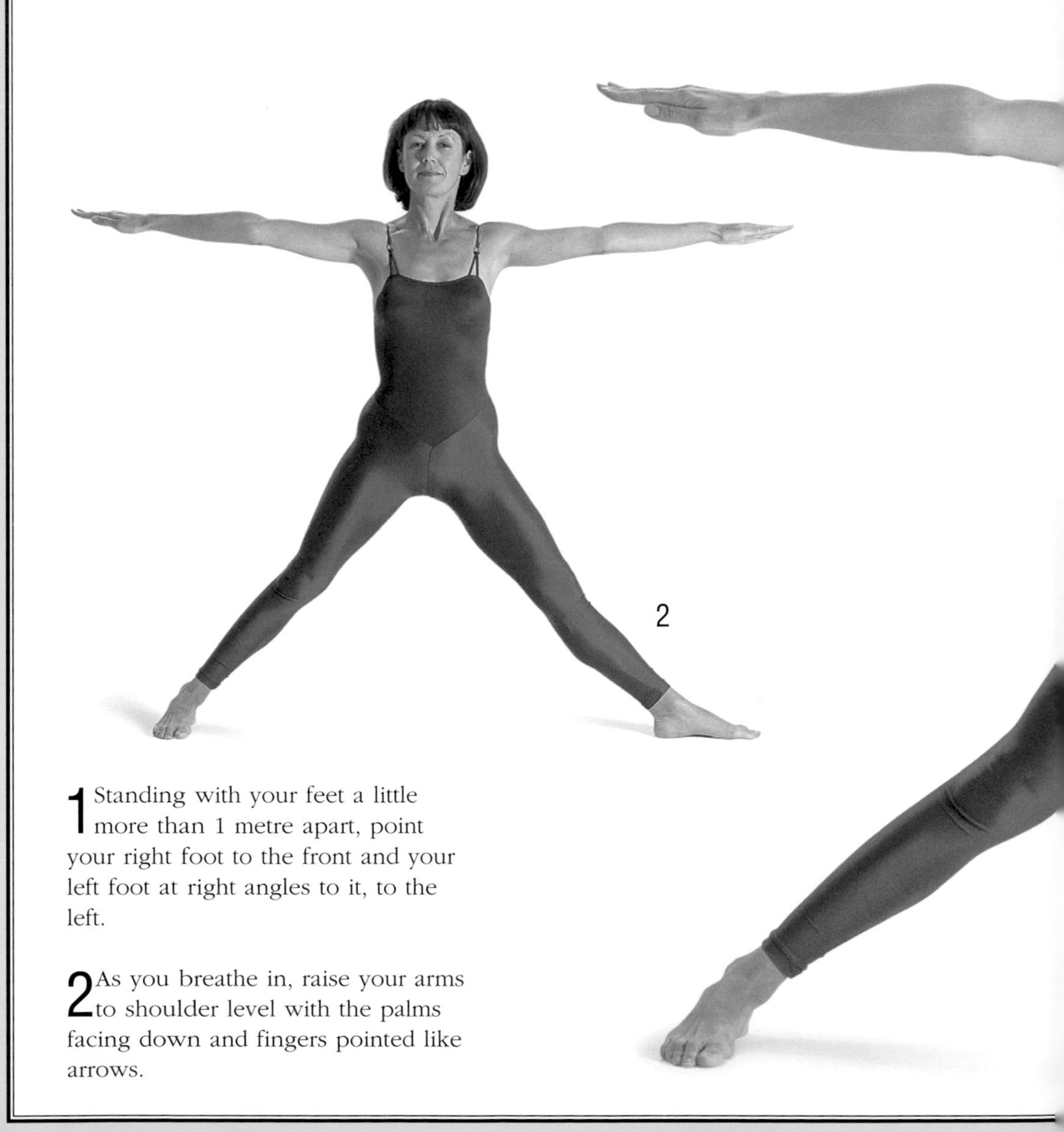

1 Standing with your feet a little more than 1 metre apart, point your right foot to the front and your left foot at right angles to it, to the left.

2 As you breathe in, raise your arms to shoulder level with the palms facing down and fingers pointed like arrows.

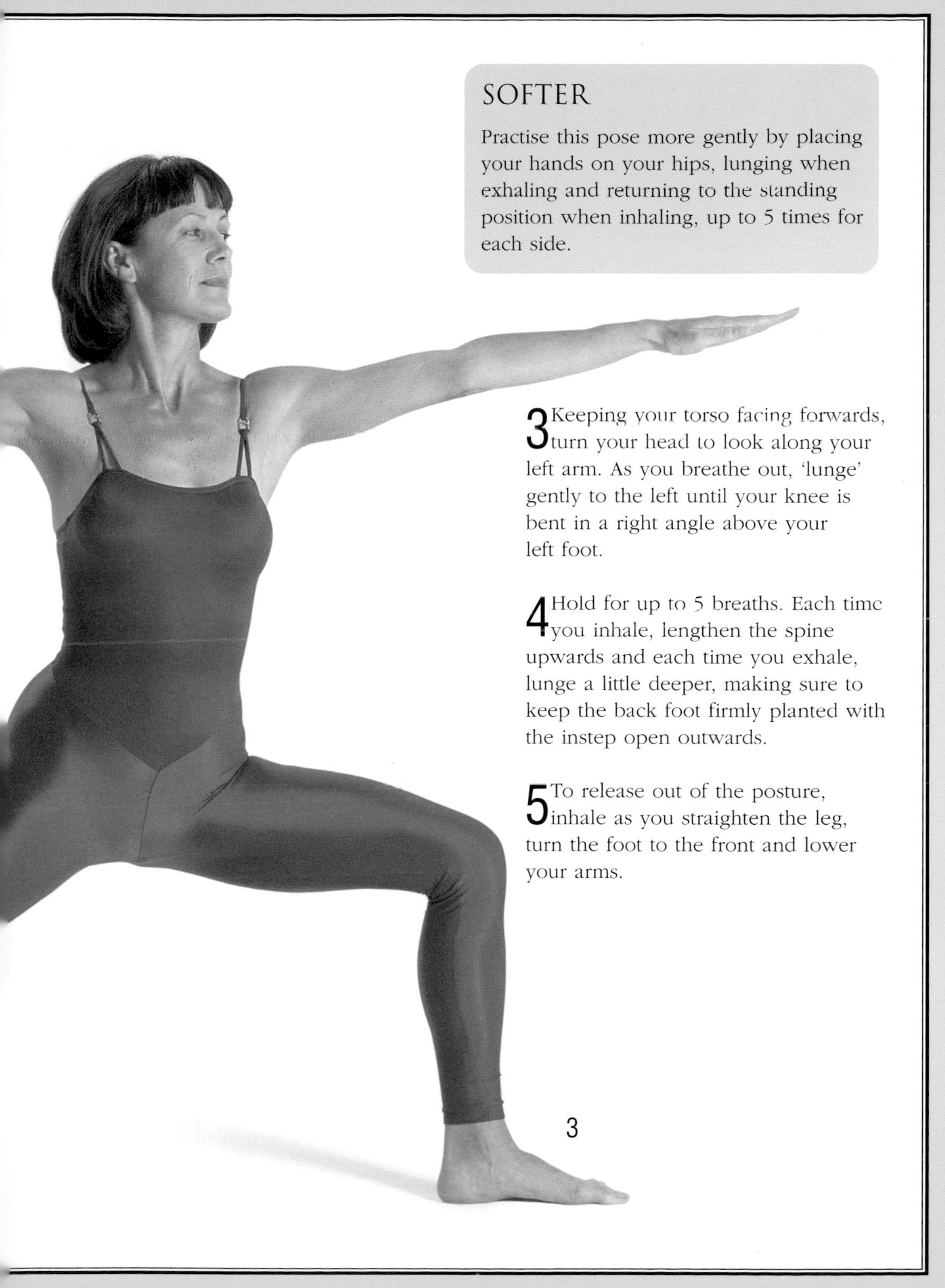

SOFTER

Practise this pose more gently by placing your hands on your hips, lunging when exhaling and returning to the standing position when inhaling, up to 5 times for each side.

3 Keeping your torso facing forwards, turn your head to look along your left arm. As you breathe out, 'lunge' gently to the left until your knee is bent in a right angle above your left foot.

4 Hold for up to 5 breaths. Each time you inhale, lengthen the spine upwards and each time you exhale, lunge a little deeper, making sure to keep the back foot firmly planted with the instep open outwards.

5 To release out of the posture, inhale as you straighten the leg, turn the foot to the front and lower your arms.

3

DANCER'S POSE

NATARAJASANA

A balancing posture that focuses the mind, the body and the breath. It works particularly to strengthen the shoulders, lower back, thighs, the flexors and the legs.

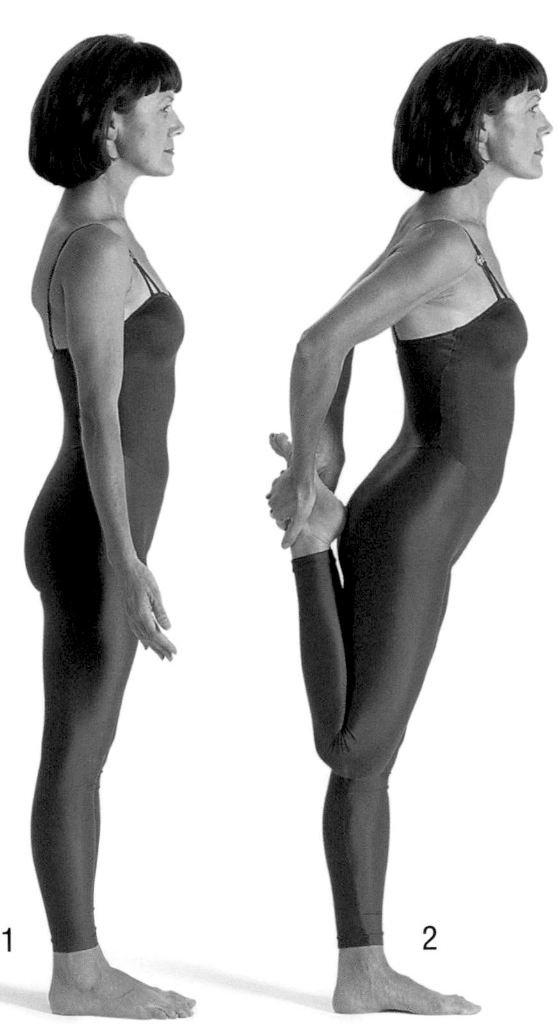

1 Stand with your feet together and your arms by your sides in the Mountain Pose (Tadasana).

2 Bend the right knee, lifting the foot up behind you. Exhale and take hold of your ankle with your right hand. Squeeze the foot into the buttock.

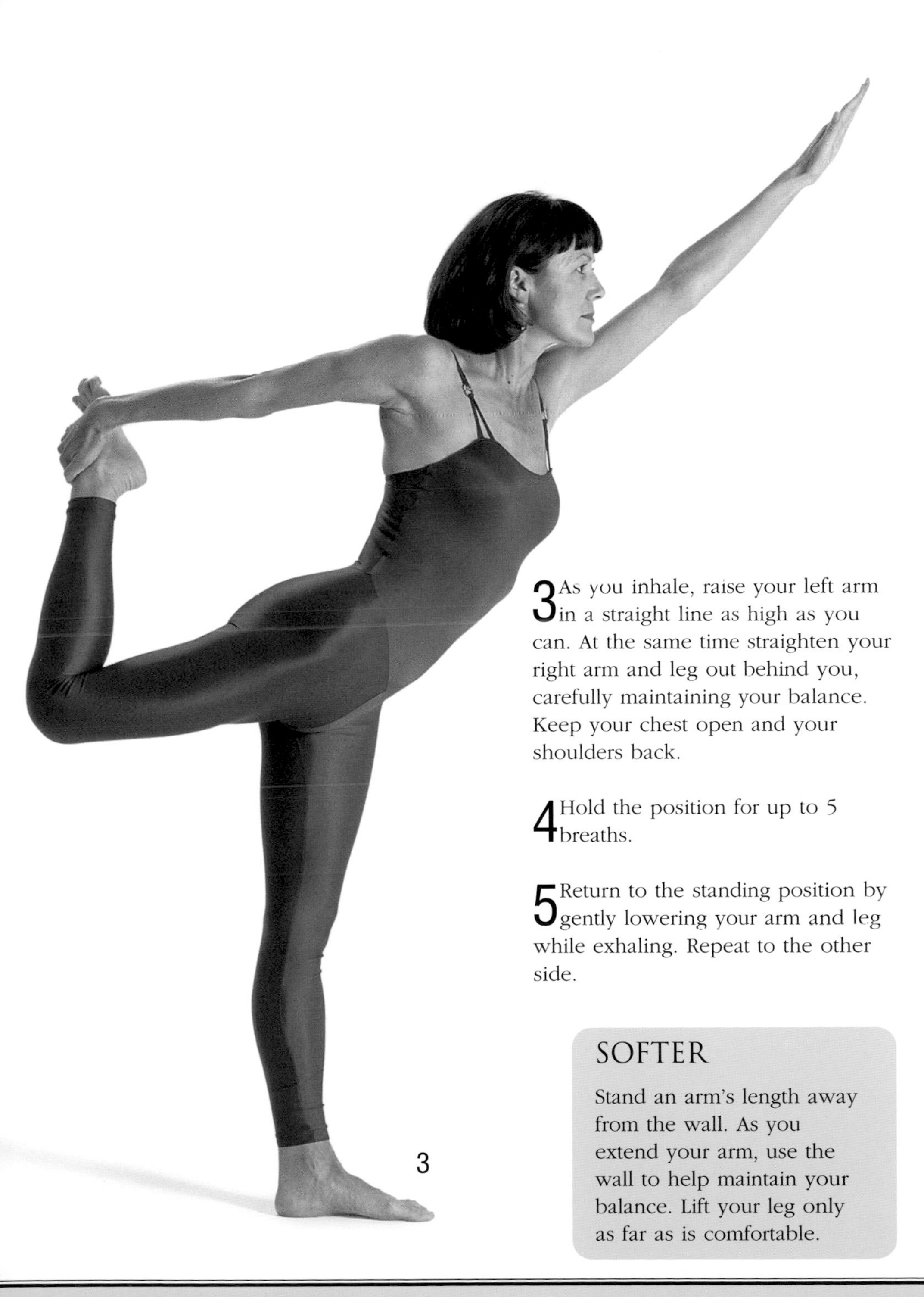

3 As you inhale, raise your left arm in a straight line as high as you can. At the same time straighten your right arm and leg out behind you, carefully maintaining your balance. Keep your chest open and your shoulders back.

4 Hold the position for up to 5 breaths.

5 Return to the standing position by gently lowering your arm and leg while exhaling. Repeat to the other side.

SOFTER

Stand an arm's length away from the wall. As you extend your arm, use the wall to help maintain your balance. Lift your leg only as far as is comfortable.

Bound Angle

Baddha Konasana

Stimulating circulation to the pelvic and reproductive organs, this sitting posture also tones the muscles in the back and releases the hips.

1 Sit with the feet drawn towards you and the soles of your feet together. Let your knees relax out and down as far as they will go.

2 Hold the toes by wrapping both hands around both feet. Lengthen your spine and straighten your arms. Allow the shoulders to relax down and back, and the chest to rise. Relax your hips and allow the soles of the feet to open.

3 Hold for up to 5 breaths. Soften and relax the hips each time you exhale.

4 Return to the starting position (knees drawn up and soles of the feet on the mat) as you gently exhale.

SOFTER

Sitting against the wall with a cushion to support your lower back, bring the soles of the feet together. Rest your hands on your knees. As you exhale, gently push down on your knees with your hands. Alternatively, lying on your back, draw the soles of your feet as far up to your groin as you can. Rest your hands on your thighs. On each exhalation allow your knees to drop down a little further towards the floor.

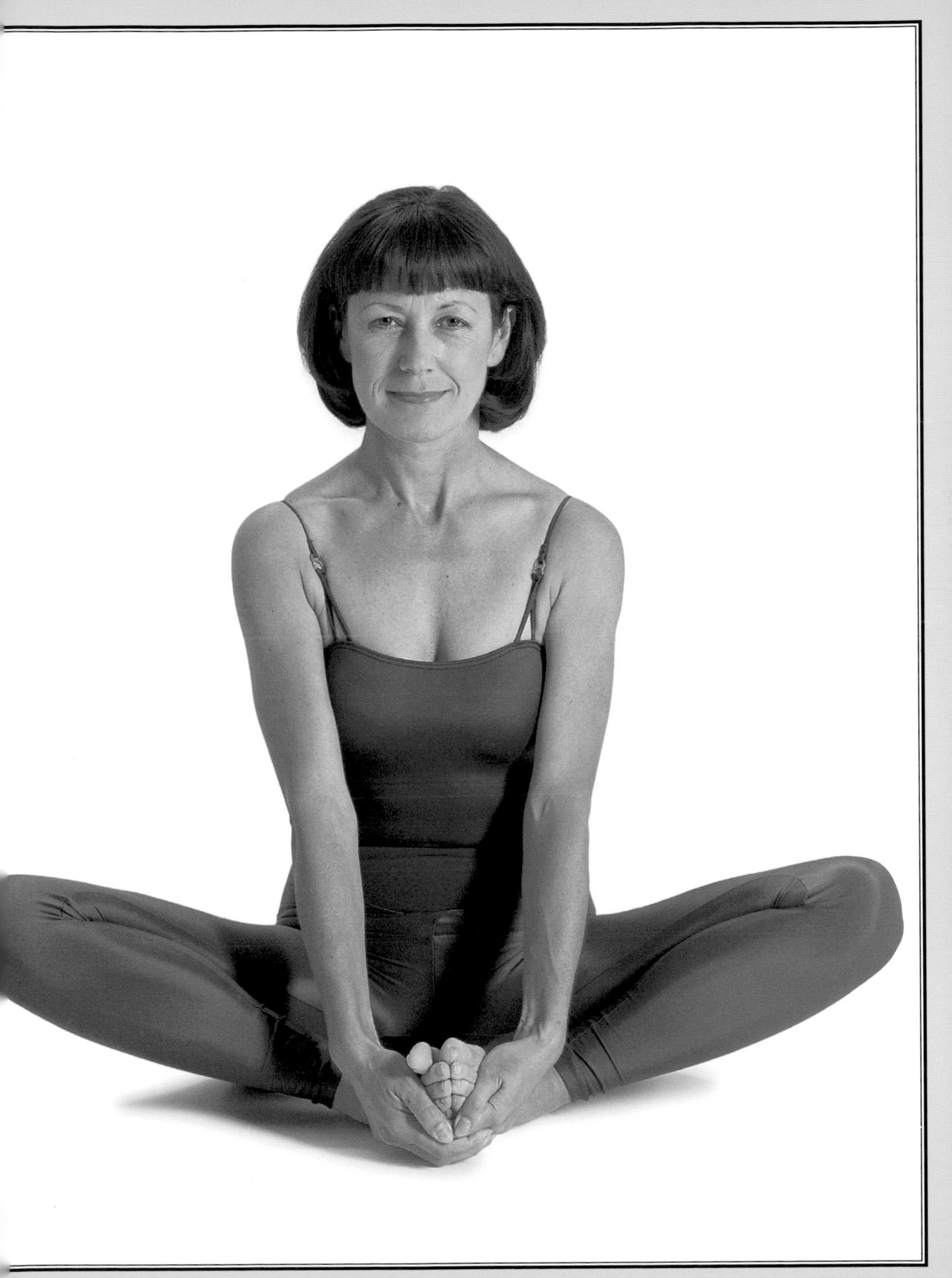

Half Bridge

Setu Bandha Sarvangasana

A strengthening and toning posture for the thighs, buttocks, and the lower and middle back.

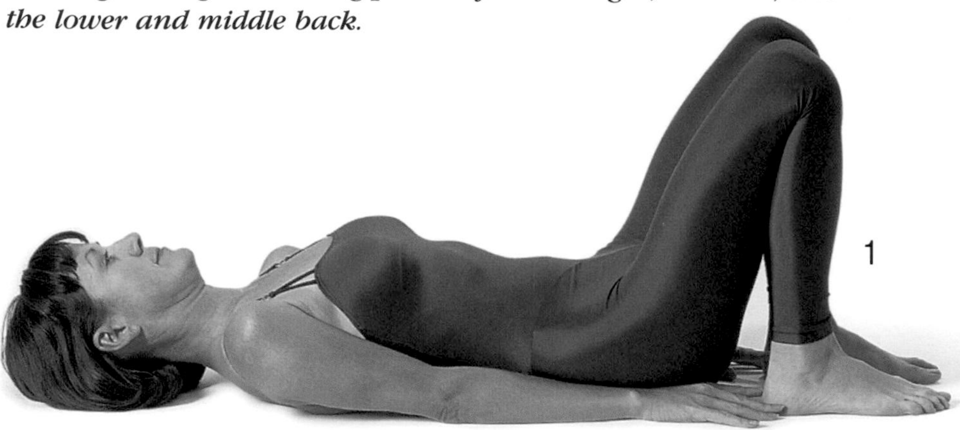

1

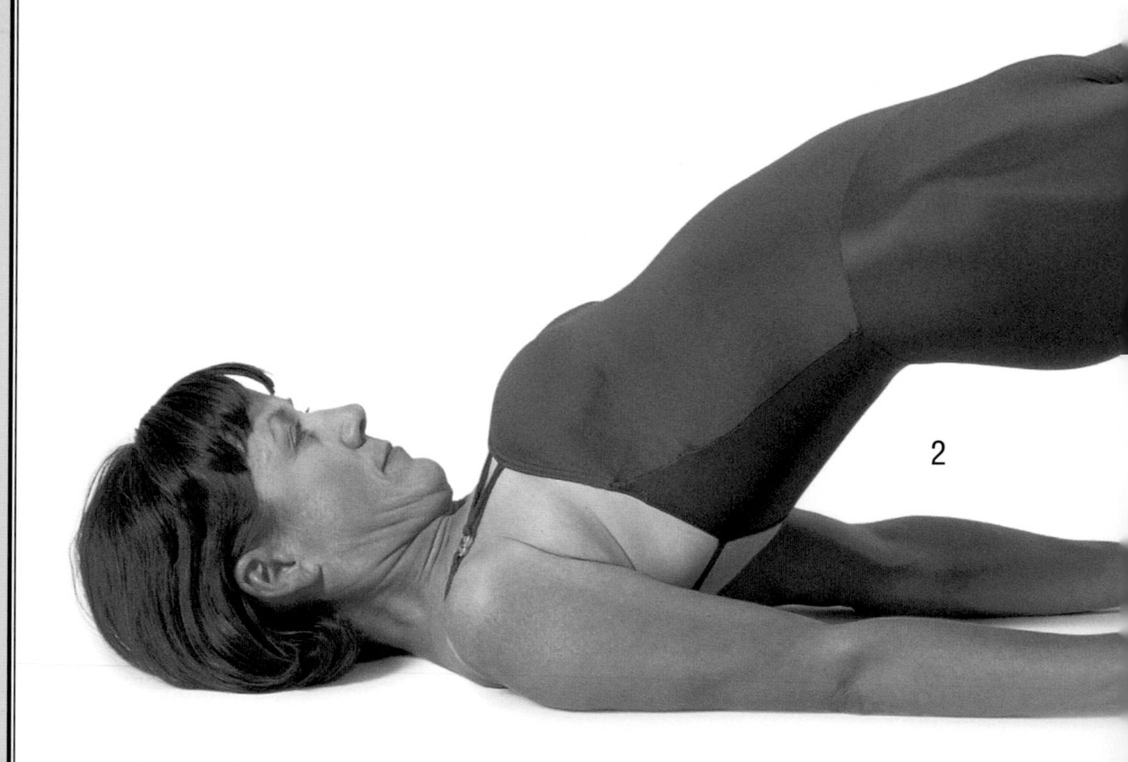

2

1 Lie flat on your back with arms at your sides. Tuck your chin in and lengthen your spine. Bend your knees and bring your feet up towards your buttocks as far as they will comfortably go. Keep your feet at hip width apart. Exhale completely.

2 Inhale as you push down on the floor with your feet, gently raising your hips, rolling your spine up slowly, one vertebra at a time. Lengthen your arms towards your ankles under your body, drawing the elbows and shoulders in.

3 Your head, neck and shoulders remain flat on the mat. Hold this position for up to 5 breaths.

4 Exhale as you lower your back one vertebra at a time.

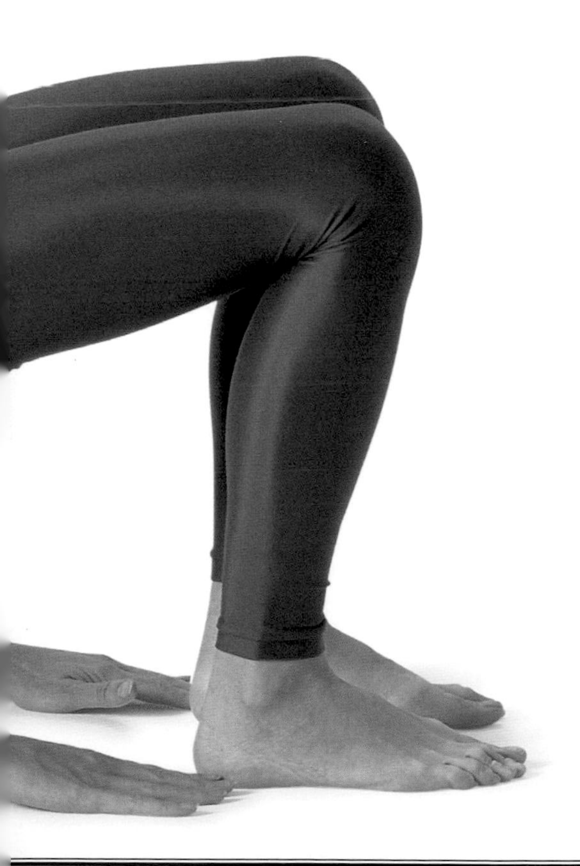

SOFTER

Leaving your arms on the floor beside you, raise your hips and chest as you inhale. Pause for a moment, then exhale as you lower your torso back to the ground. Repeat up to 5 times.

SHOULDER STAND

SARVANGASANA

This inverted pose stimulates blood circulation and increases the oxygen supply to the head. It also stimulates the thyroid gland, and strengthens the back and abdominal muscles.

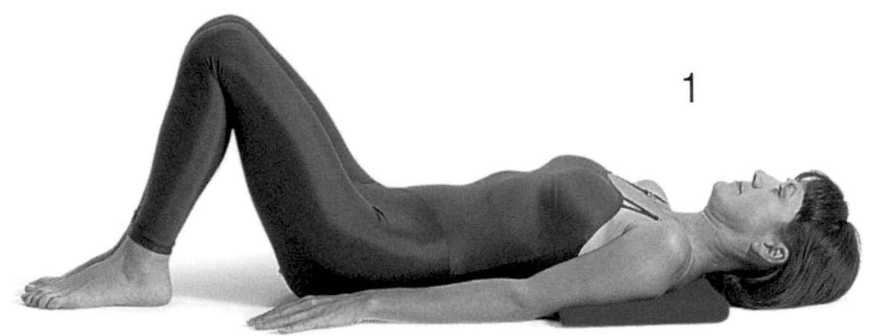

1 Lying on the floor with your legs and feet together and your arms by your sides, exhale completely.

2 Inhale as you draw your knees up to your chest and exhale as you continue to roll your knees up to your forehead. Place your hands as far up your back to your shoulder blades as you can.

3 Maintaining your balance, carefully extend your legs to the vertical position. Keep your eyes open and look up at your feet. Hold for up to 5 breaths.

4 To come down, exhale and gently bend your knees until they are touching your forehead again. Lower your hands to the floor and use them for support as you roll your torso down. Inhale as you straighten your legs along the mat.

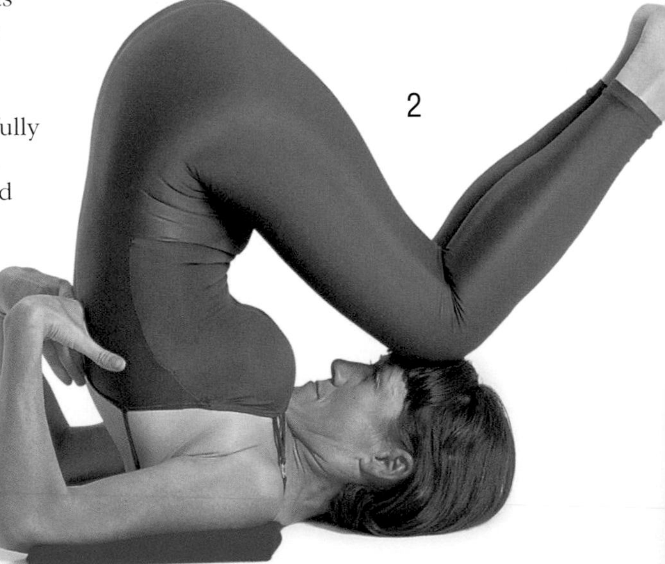

SOFTER

Using the wall to help you achieve the inverted pose.

1 Lying on the floor, bring your hips close to the wall. Align your body so that your feet rest on the wall, slightly above the height of your bent knees. Your arms should be by your sides and your chin tucked in slightly. Exhale completely.

2 Inhale and push against the wall with your feet, raising your hips as high as you can. Place your hands in the small of your back, thumbs turned in towards the spine, and fingers pointing out around your hips. Exhale.

3 Breathe in and slowly walk your feet up the wall as far as you can. Hold in this position for up to 5 breaths. Breathe out and walk your feet gently down again.

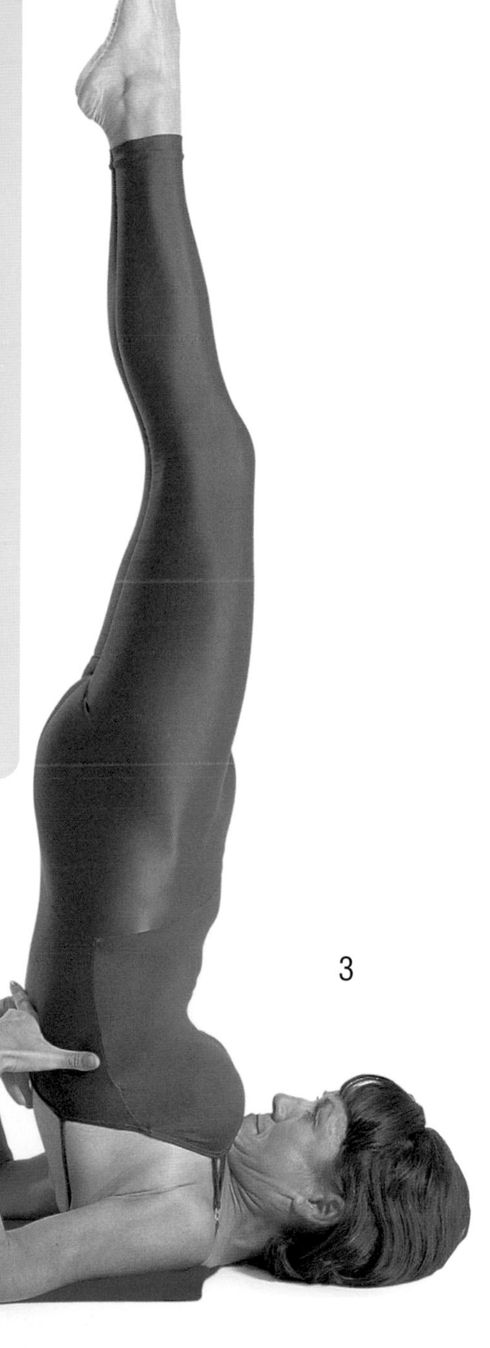

Fish Pose

Matsyasana

The fish pose is a lovely counter pose to the shoulder stand. It encourages good posture, opens the chest and strengthens the neck muscles.

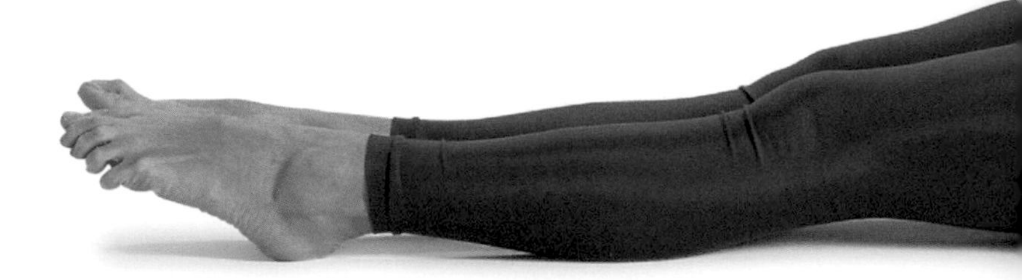

1 Lie flat on your back with your knees bent and your knees and feet together. Push down on the mat with your feet and lift your buttocks. Place your hands palms downward under your buttocks. The elbows should be tucked in under the back. Lower your buttocks onto your hands.

2 Exhale as you straighten your legs along the mat. As you inhale, push your elbows into the mat, and bend your arms so that your chest rises. Keep your legs and buttocks on the floor, and allow your head to drop gently back.

3 Breathe deeply and comfortably into the expanded chest for up to 5 breaths.

4 To come out of the posture, lift your head slightly, relax your elbows and breathe out as you lower your back to the floor.

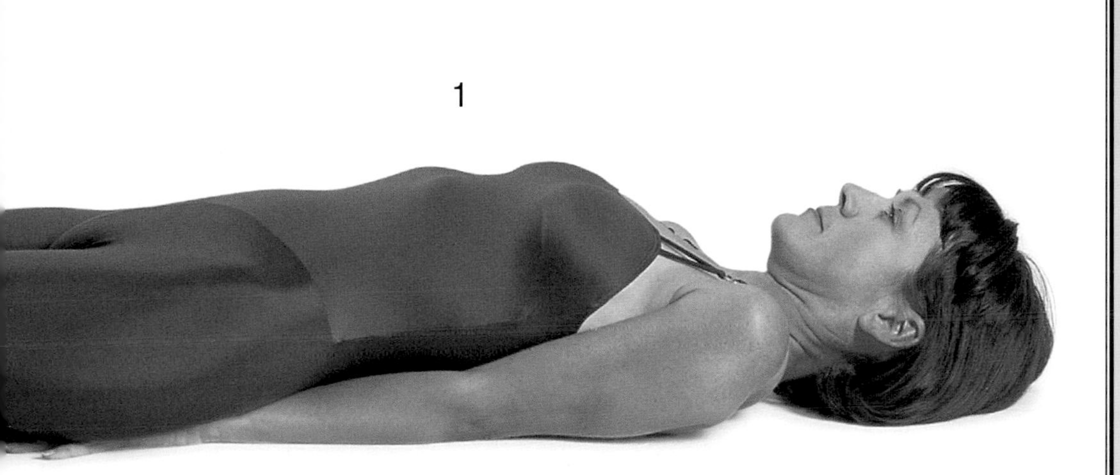

2

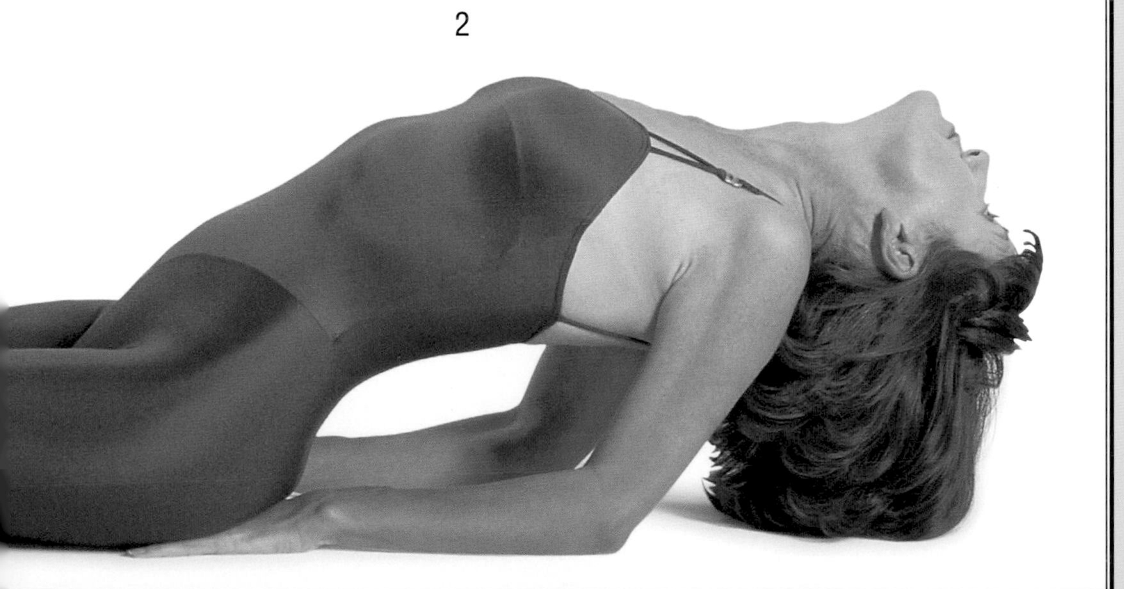

TWISTING POSE

MATSYENDRASANA

A practice that helps with strengthening and toning the shoulders, spine and buttocks, and massaging the internal organs.

1 Sit with your legs crossed so that the left foot is in front of the right. Push your sitting bones back and lengthen your spine.

2 Exhale and bring your left foot over your right knee.

3 Roll your left shoulder back and place your left hand on the mat behind the buttocks at the base of your spine. Hug your left knee with your right arm. Hold the position for up to 5 breaths. On each inbreath extend the spine upward. On every outbreath, twist gently to look over your left shoulder.

4 Return to the sitting position with legs crossed. Bend your torso forward over your crossed legs as you exhale. As you inhale, straighten the torso again.

5 Change your leg position so that the right foot is now in front of the left and repeat the instructions twisting to the opposite side.

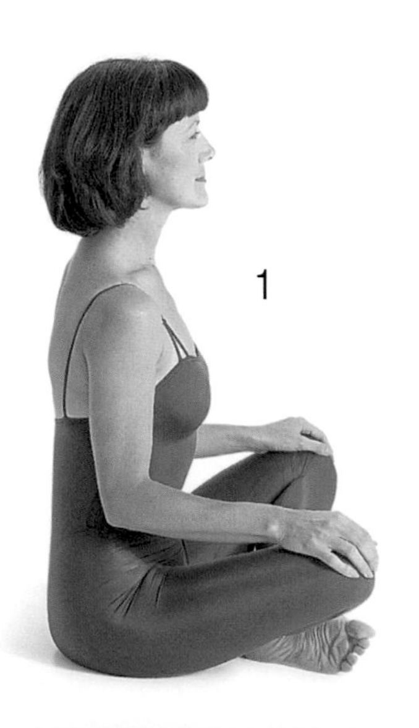

1

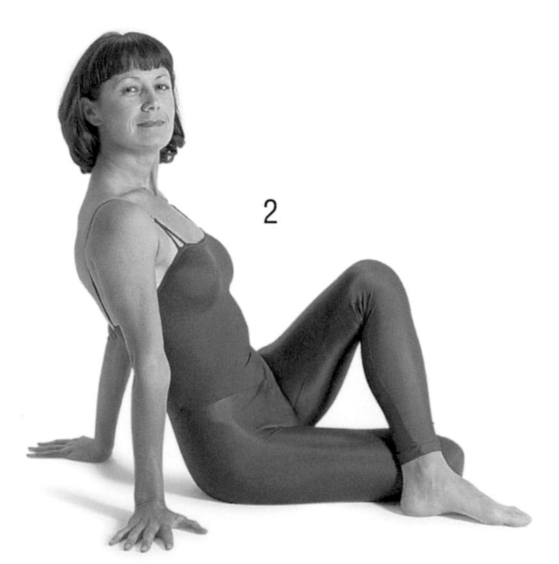

2

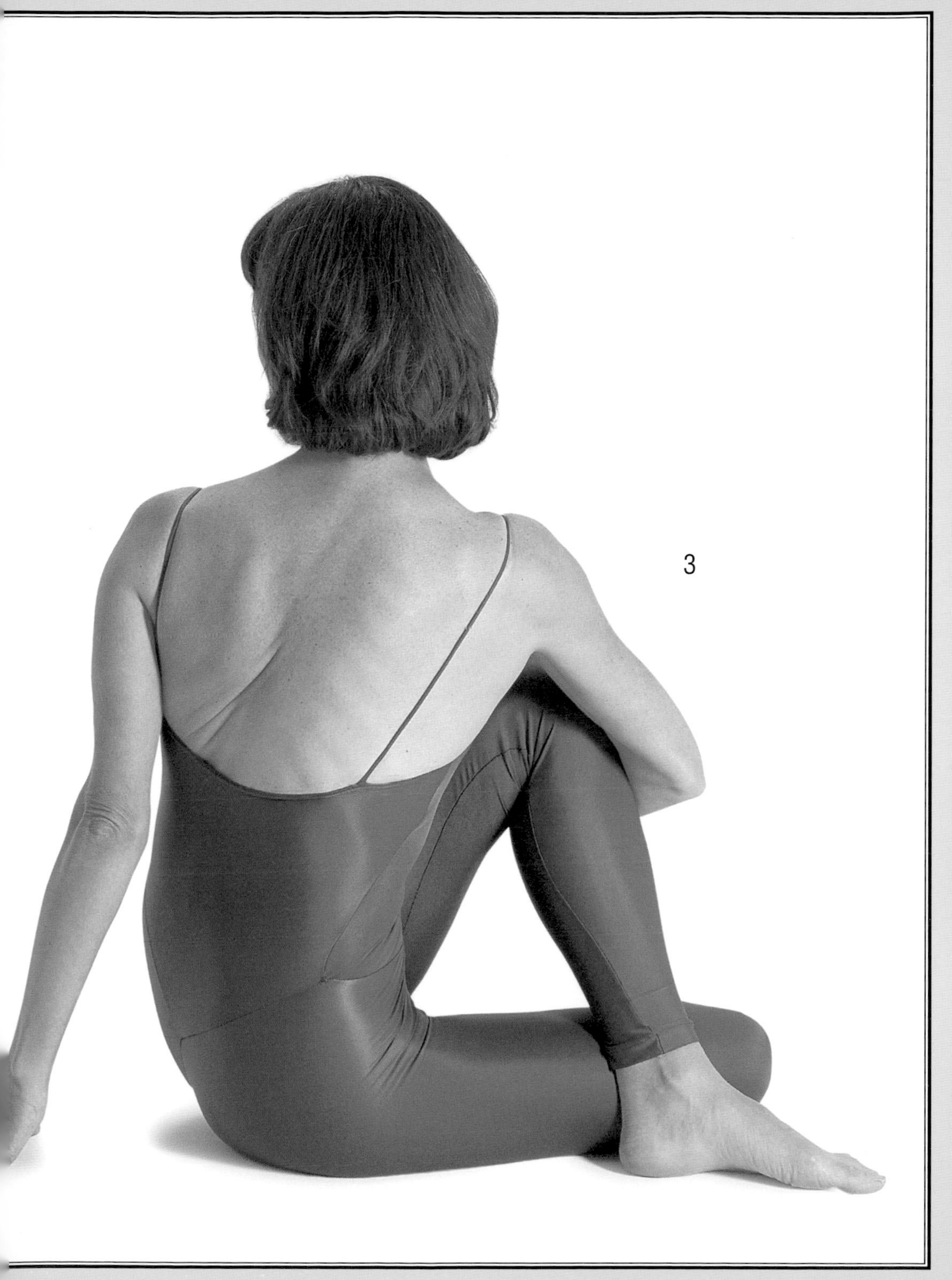
3

Twisting II

A softer alternative to the previous exercises.

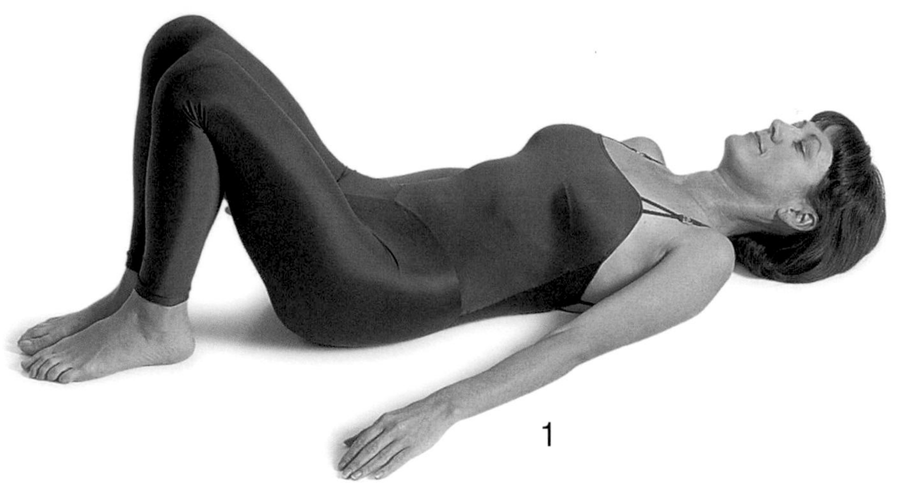

1

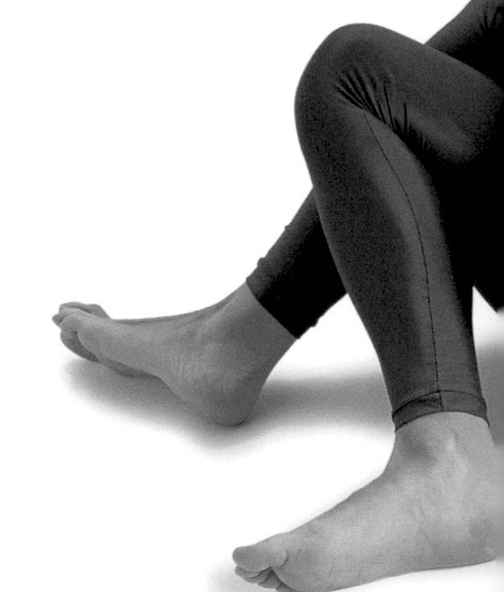

1 Lie on your back with your knees bent and your feet on the floor. Place your arms a little away from your sides with the palms facing down.

2 Lift the left leg and cross it over the right knee.

3 Exhale as you roll both legs to the right and roll your head gently to the left. It is important to keep your chin tucked in and both shoulders on the floor.

4 Hold the position for up to 5 breaths. Inhale as you roll back to the centre and uncross your legs. Repeat to the other side.

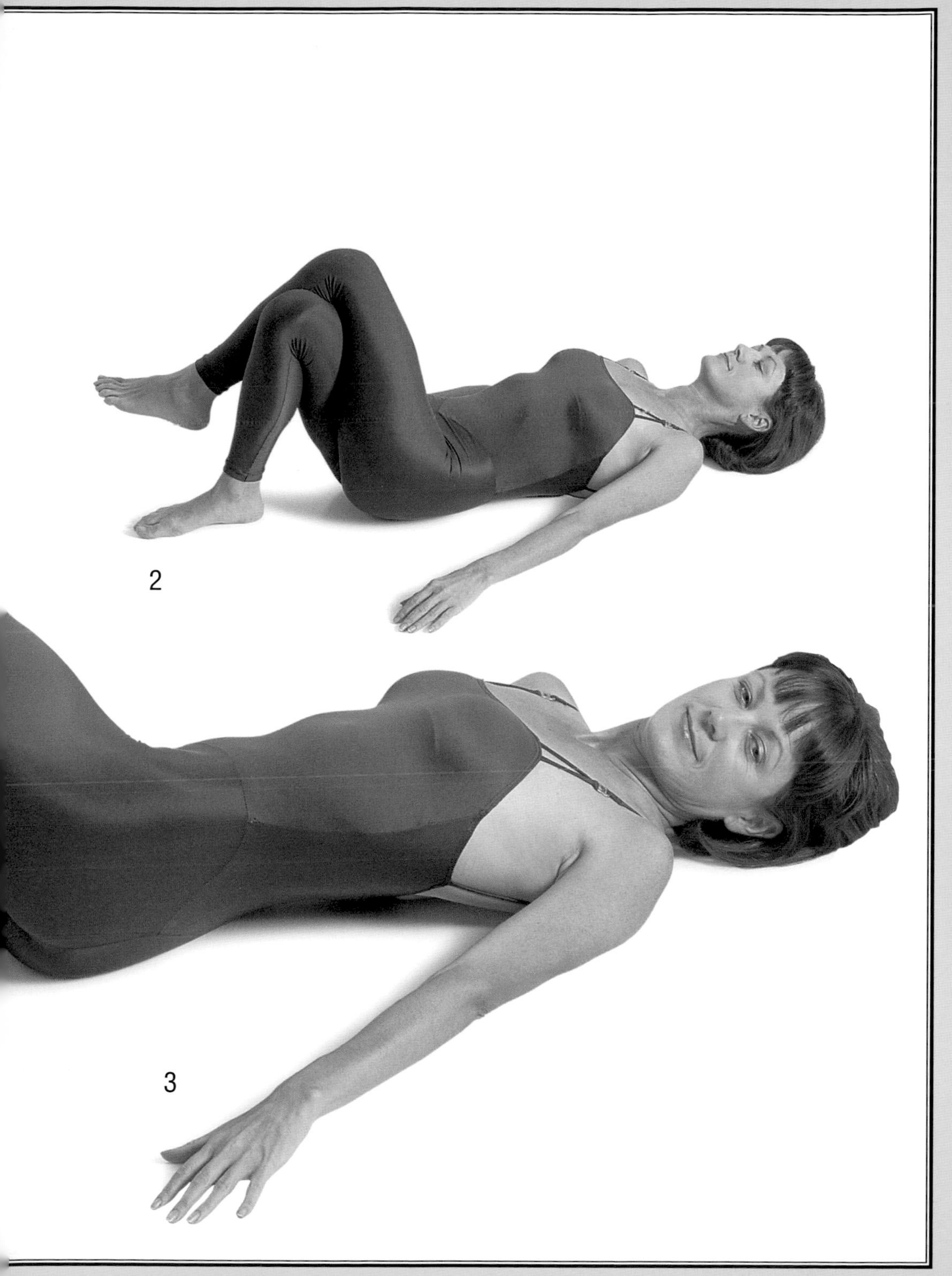
2
3

Hand to Foot

Ubhaya Padangusthasana

This pose works to open the back, lengthen the hamstrings and strengthen the shoulders. It is an excellent preparation for the Corpse Pose which follows it.

1 Sitting on the mat, draw your knees towards your chest, keeping your feet together on the floor. Reaching around your legs, grasp each big toe in the yoga hook (the first two fingers curled around the big toe).

2 Draw your knees towards your chest and lift your heels off the floor. Balancing on your sitting bones, with your eyes focused on your feet, carefully raise your legs. Tuck your chin in slightly, straighten your back and slowly push your heels away from your body.

3 Hold the position for up to 5 breaths. Release gently out of the posture on the exhaling breath as you bend your knees and lower your feet.

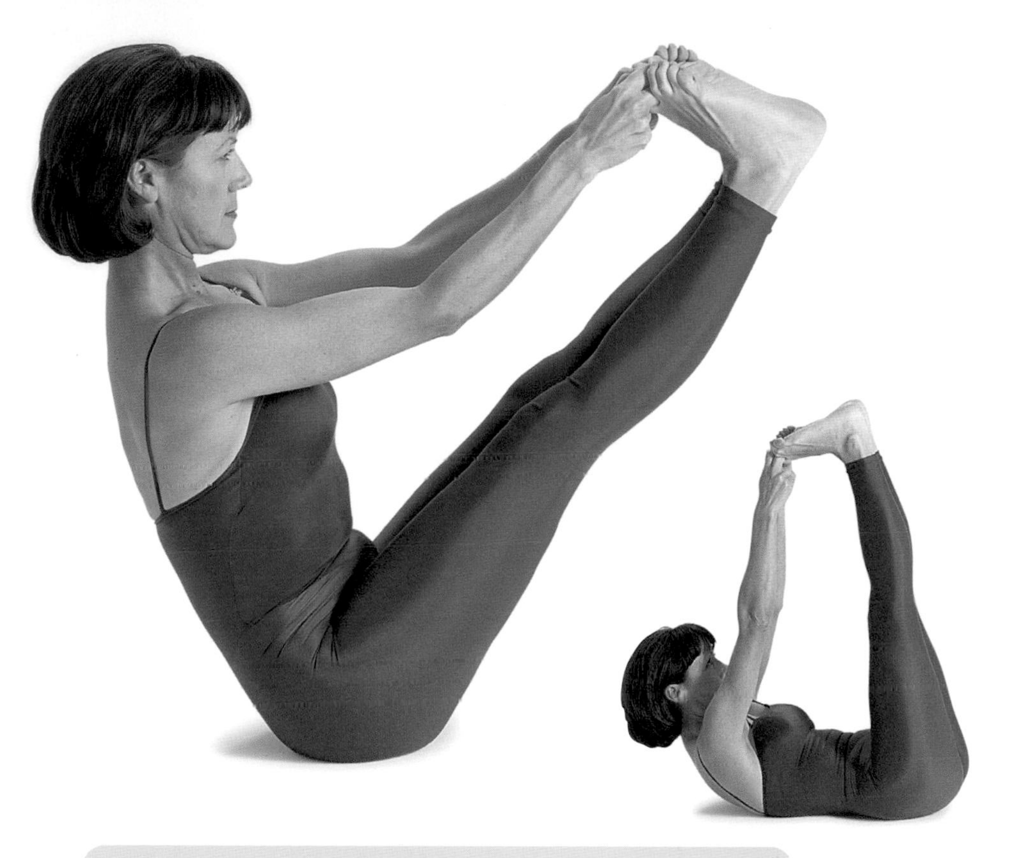

SOFTER

1 Lie on your back with your knees drawn up to your chest. Reaching around your legs, hold your big toes in the yoga hook (see above). As you breathe out, tuck your chin in and lift your head towards your knees.

2 Inhale as you push your hips into the floor, and straighten your legs so that your feet reach directly upwards. Keep your head and shoulders off the floor and your chin tucked in.

3 Hold the position for up to 5 breaths. To release out of the posture, allow the knees to bend, relax your arms and return to the lying position.

Alternatively, follow the softer directions above, but hold the calves rather than the toes.

CORPSE POSE II

SAVASANA

In the last posture of the sequence, we return to the Corpse Pose which completely relaxes both the mind and the body.

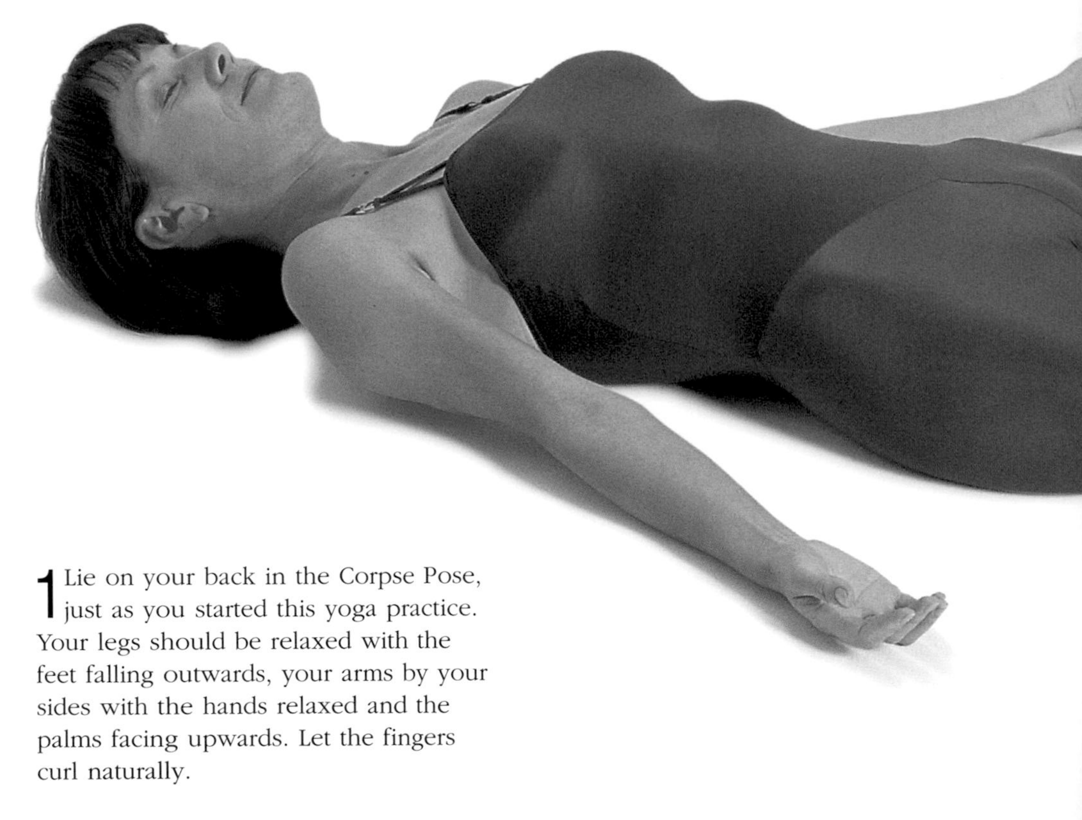

1 Lie on your back in the Corpse Pose, just as you started this yoga practice. Your legs should be relaxed with the feet falling outwards, your arms by your sides with the hands relaxed and the palms facing upwards. Let the fingers curl naturally.

2 Close your eyes, tuck your chin in a little, spread your shoulders and lengthen your spine.

Now just let go, surrender and soften the face. Let the eyes, the brow and the ears melt back into the mat. Soften the jaw, unclench your teeth and let your tongue be soft in your mouth. Continue this softness down your throat and neck. Allow your shoulders to melt into the mat, relax your spine and soften your back muscles. Feel the lower back melt into the mat and let the hips open. Soften the buttocks, the abdomen and the thighs and let this softness continue down the legs, into the feet and the toes.

Completely surrender your body and let your thoughts float away like clouds. Allow yourself to relax completely for at least 5 minutes.

When you are ready, roll onto your right side and rest for a moment in this position as you bring your awareness back to the everyday world. Slowly come up to the sitting position and give yourself a few more moments, to feel completely at peace, positive about your life and your yoga practice.

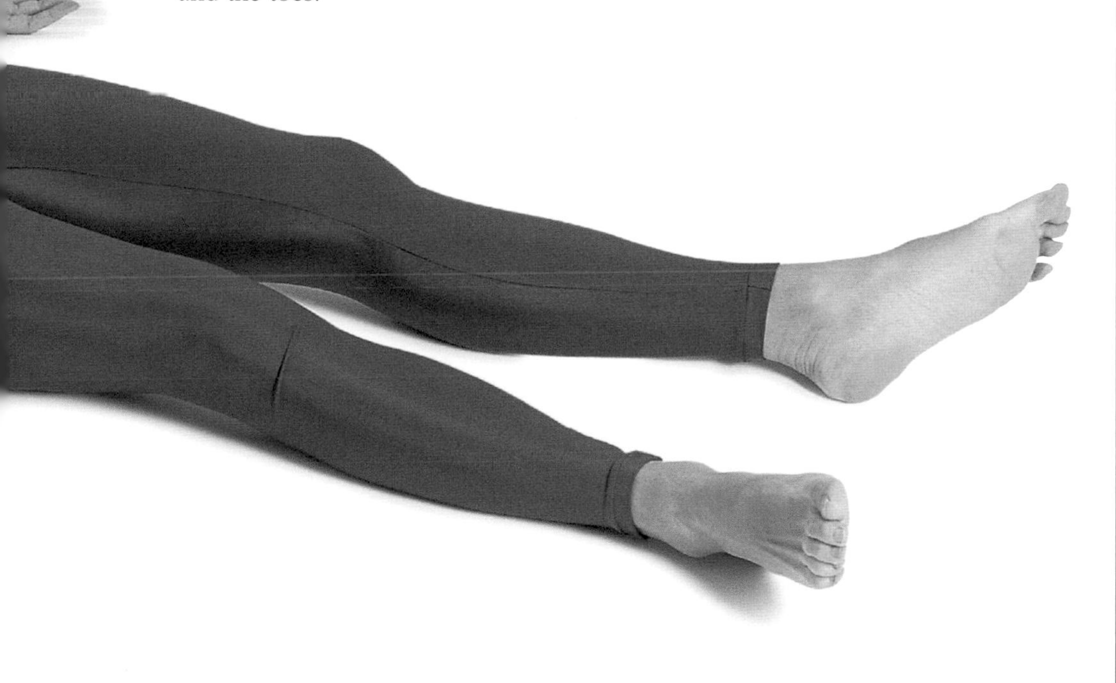

Sun Salutation

Suyra Namaskar

Begin by standing on your mat in the Mountain Pose (Tadasana). Bring your feet together (toes and ankles touching) with your arms by your sides. Lengthen your spine upwards from the tip of the tail bone to the crown of the head. Inhale deeply.

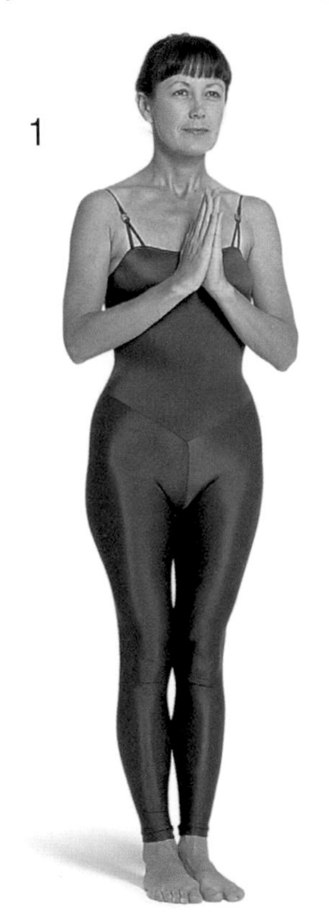

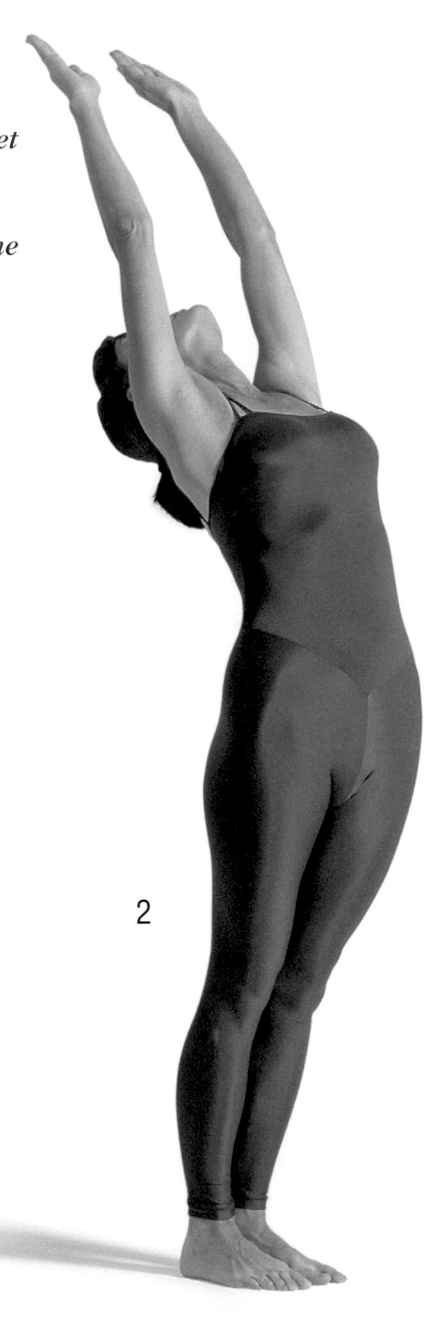

1 Exhale and bring the hands together in the 'prayer' position.

2 Inhale as you stretch your arms up beside your head, lengthening and arching your spine.

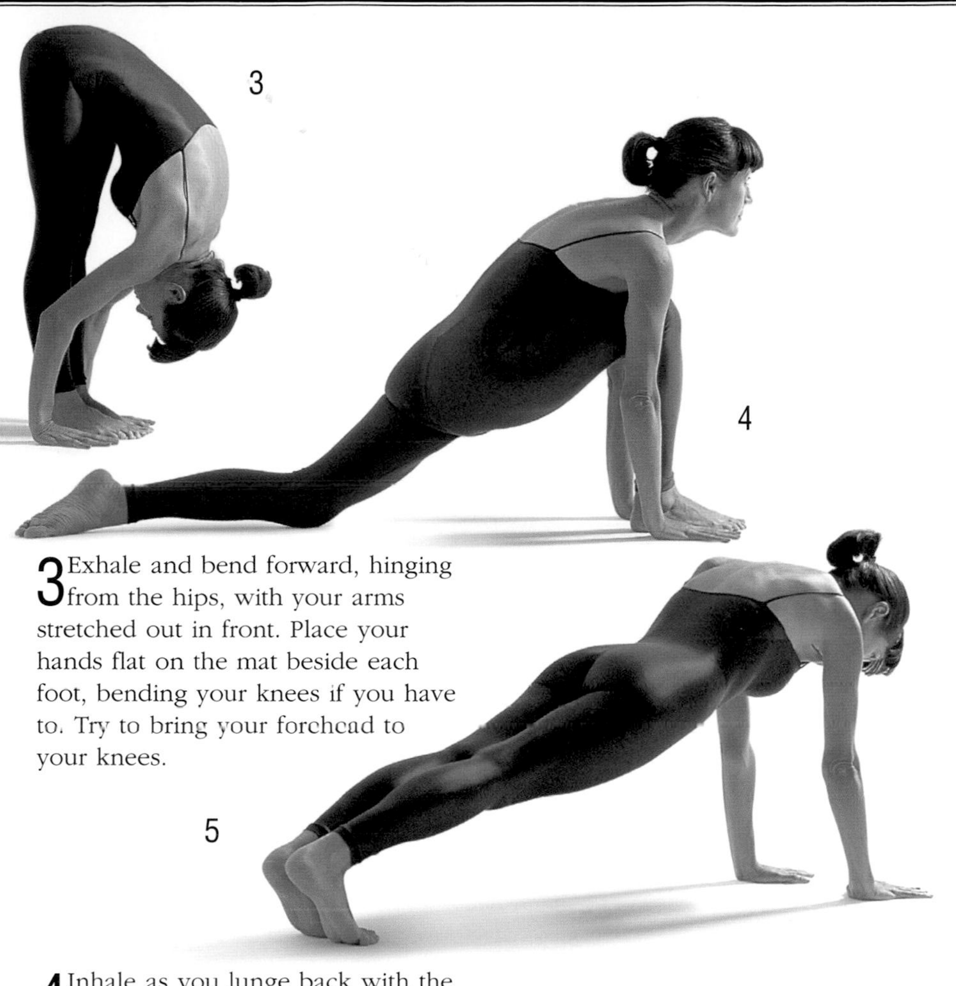

3 Exhale and bend forward, hinging from the hips, with your arms stretched out in front. Place your hands flat on the mat beside each foot, bending your knees if you have to. Try to bring your forehead to your knees.

4 Inhale as you lunge back with the left foot as far as possible. Place your left knee on the mat, drawing the chest and the head upwards.

5 Hold your breath and bring both feet (with the toes tucked under) back into 'pole' position so that the body is in a straight line from head to heels, with your hands under your shoulders.

6 Maintaining the position of your hands and keeping your hips up, exhale as you bring your knees, chest and chin down to the mat.

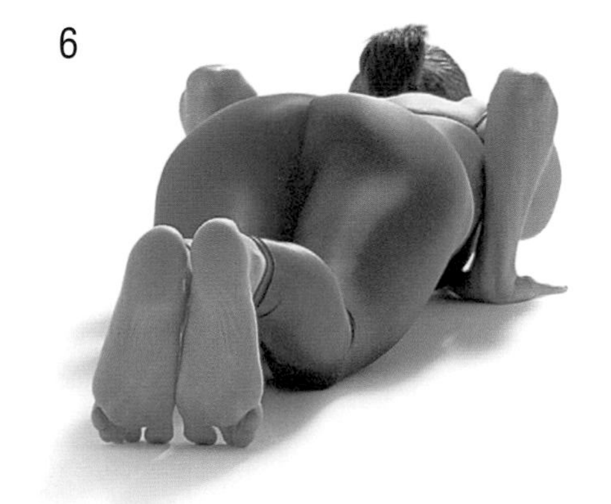

Sun Salutation

(Continued)

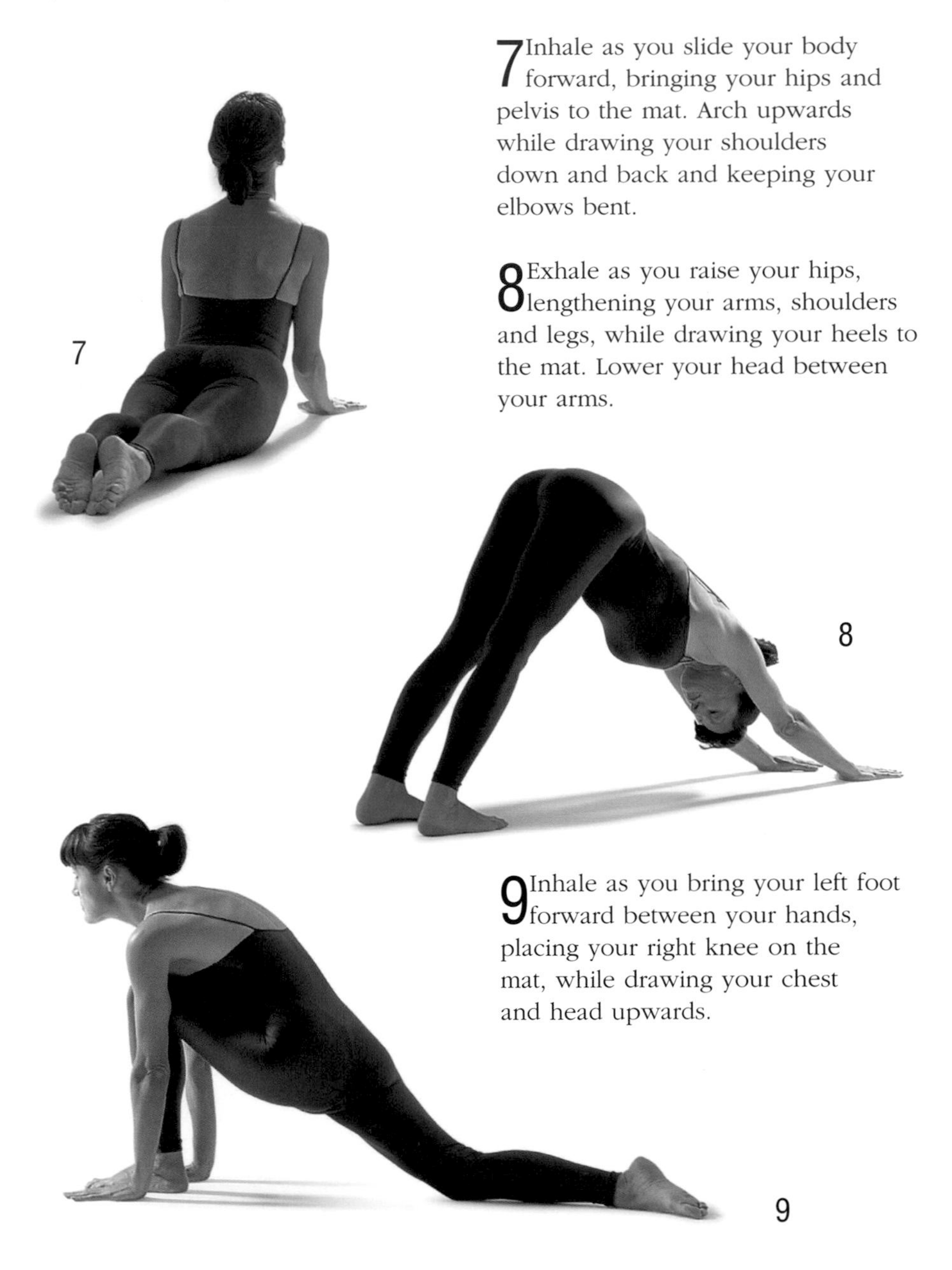

7 Inhale as you slide your body forward, bringing your hips and pelvis to the mat. Arch upwards while drawing your shoulders down and back and keeping your elbows bent.

8 Exhale as you raise your hips, lengthening your arms, shoulders and legs, while drawing your heels to the mat. Lower your head between your arms.

9 Inhale as you bring your left foot forward between your hands, placing your right knee on the mat, while drawing your chest and head upwards.

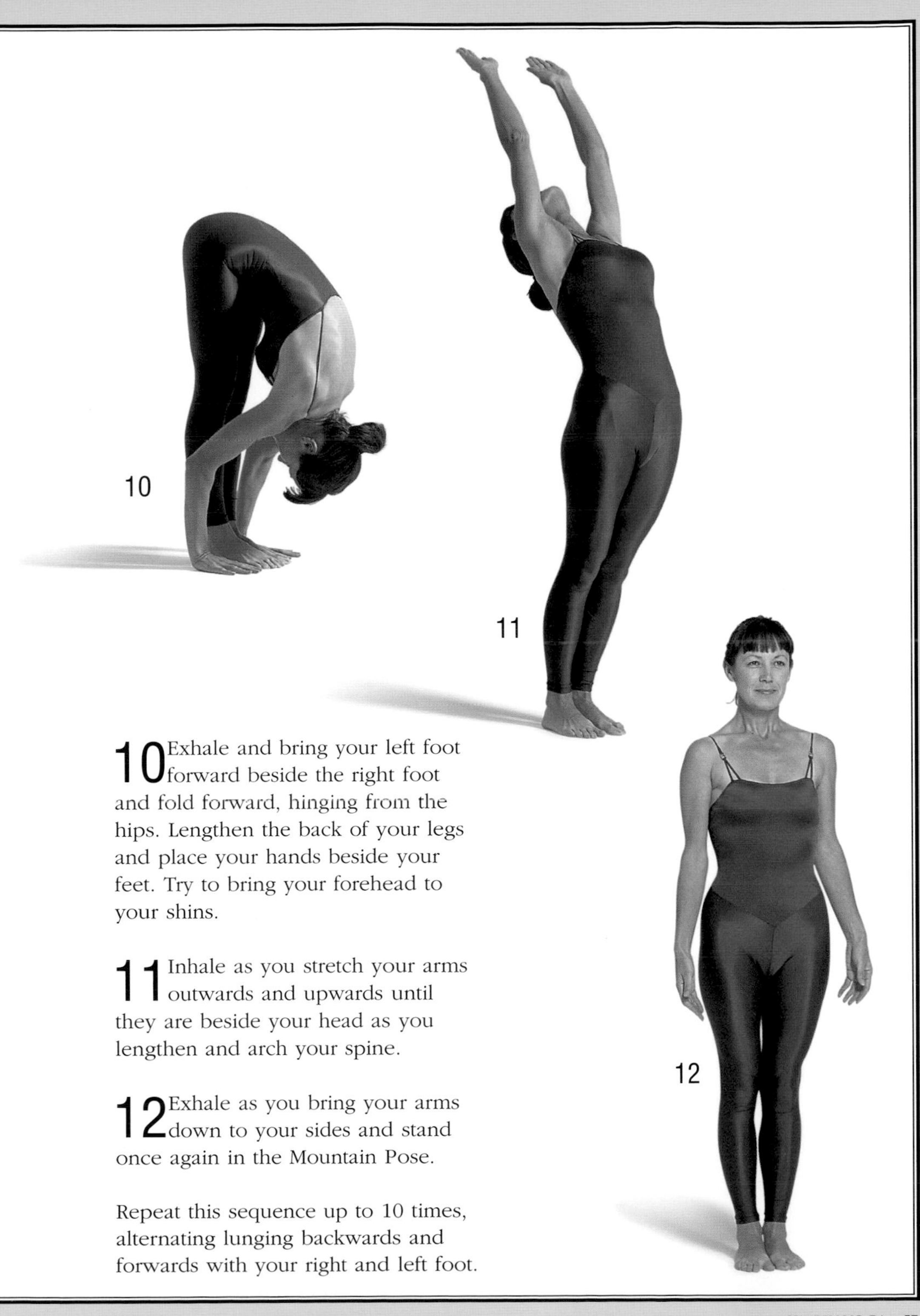

10 Exhale and bring your left foot forward beside the right foot and fold forward, hinging from the hips. Lengthen the back of your legs and place your hands beside your feet. Try to bring your forehead to your shins.

11 Inhale as you stretch your arms outwards and upwards until they are beside your head as you lengthen and arch your spine.

12 Exhale as you bring your arms down to your sides and stand once again in the Mountain Pose.

Repeat this sequence up to 10 times, alternating lunging backwards and forwards with your right and left foot.

Saluting The Sun

Complete Sequence

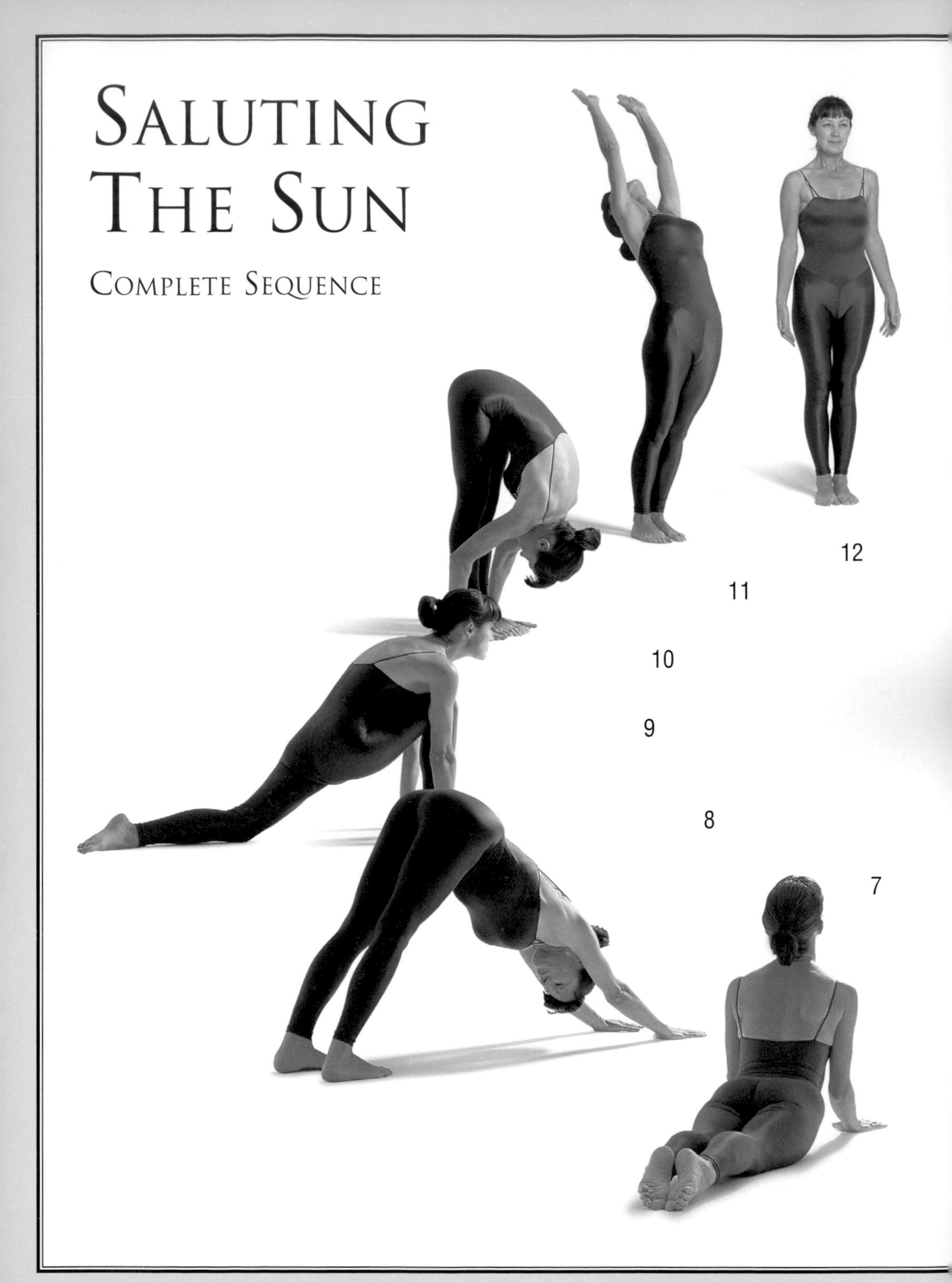

SALUTATION

The Sun Salutation consists of twelve postures giving various vertebral movements to the spinal column. It brings great flexibility and strength to the spine and the limbs. It also helps to regulate the breath and focus the mind. This sequence can be practised on its own or as an alternative to the previous sequences described.

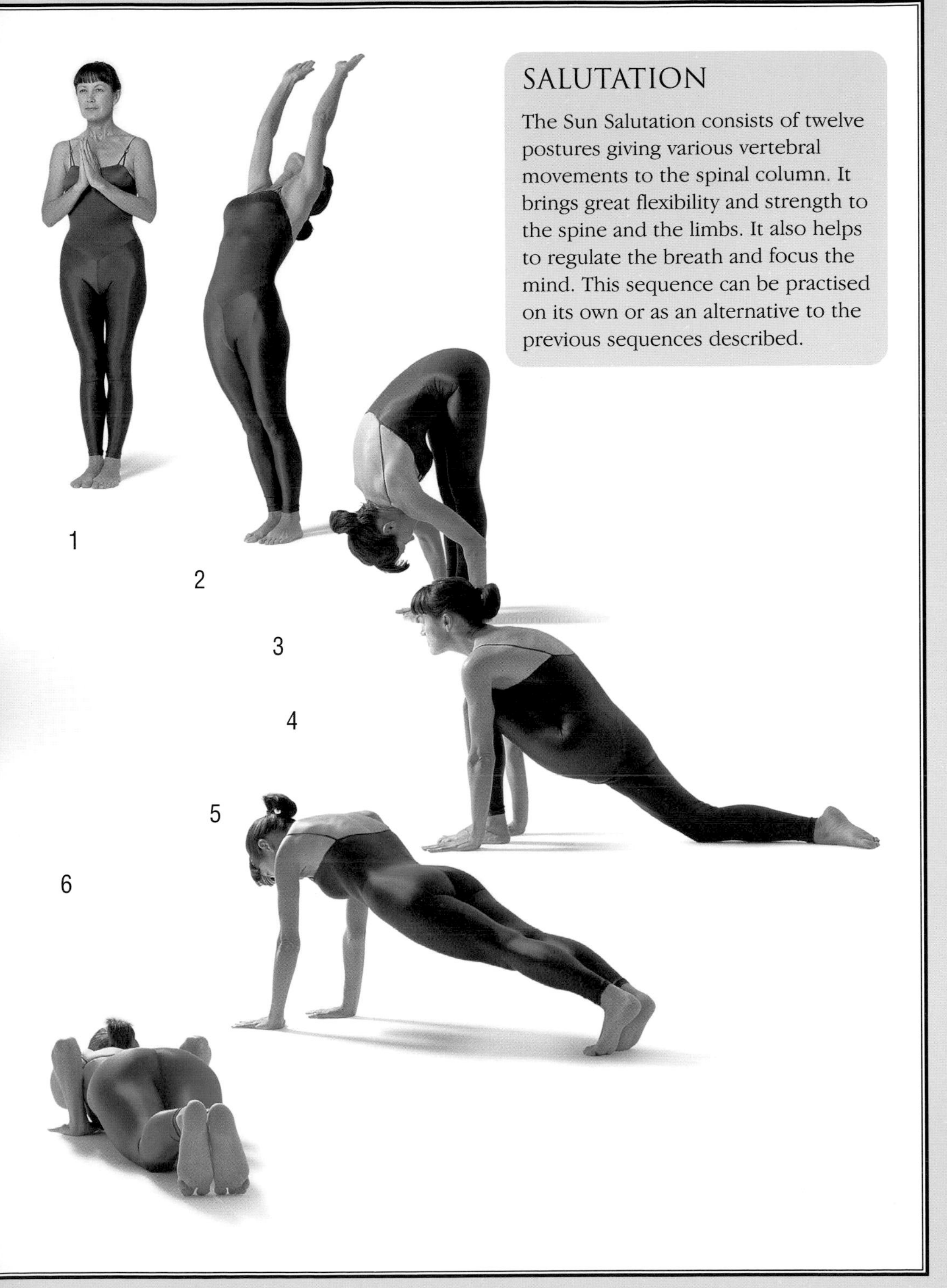

MEDITATION

CALMING THE MIND

A calming practice that brings increased mental clarity, increased energy levels and greater capacity for contentment.

The word meditation is naturally associated with the practice of Yoga. It describes a state of inner stillness, a feeling of balance and peace that, with regular practice, will radiate from one's daily routine into the everyday world of our busy lives. It is not the purpose of this book to explore meditation in any depth, but the following simple practice is one you might like to try while your body is feeling relaxed and alert at the end of the posture sequence. Or it can be practised on its own.

1 Make sure your surroundings are comfortably warm and quiet. Allow 5 to 10 minutes at first. Gradually increase the time to 20 minutes or more, as you feel able.

2 Sit comfortably with a straight back and with legs crossed. Rest the hands lightly on the knees or the thighs. Sitting on a firm pillow or a folded blanket can help you to keep your spine straight.

3 Close your eyes and gently bring your attention inward, away from the external world. Soften your face. Tuck your chin in. Relax your neck and shoulder muscles. Breathe gently and evenly.

4 Bring your awareness to any thoughts that come into your mind. See if you can simply observe them, letting them come, and letting them go, without following them. It's as if your mind is a beautiful, clear blue sky, and your thoughts are small, white clouds passing across it. Be patient with yourself. Your mind is used to getting its own way; some days your thoughts may be many and your mind might seem like an overcast sky. By quietly observing the thoughts they will slow down and become fewer. Enjoy the spaces between the thoughts. Allow that sense of peace and wellbeing to expand as your mind clears and becomes quiet.

SOFTER

Sit on the floor against a wall with your back straight and legs either crossed or outstretched. Place a small cushion in the small of your back. OR – Sit on an upright chair with your back straight and your feet placed flat on the floor directly under your knees. Push your buttocks into the back of the chair. Use a folded blanket under the feet if your heels do not touch the floor.

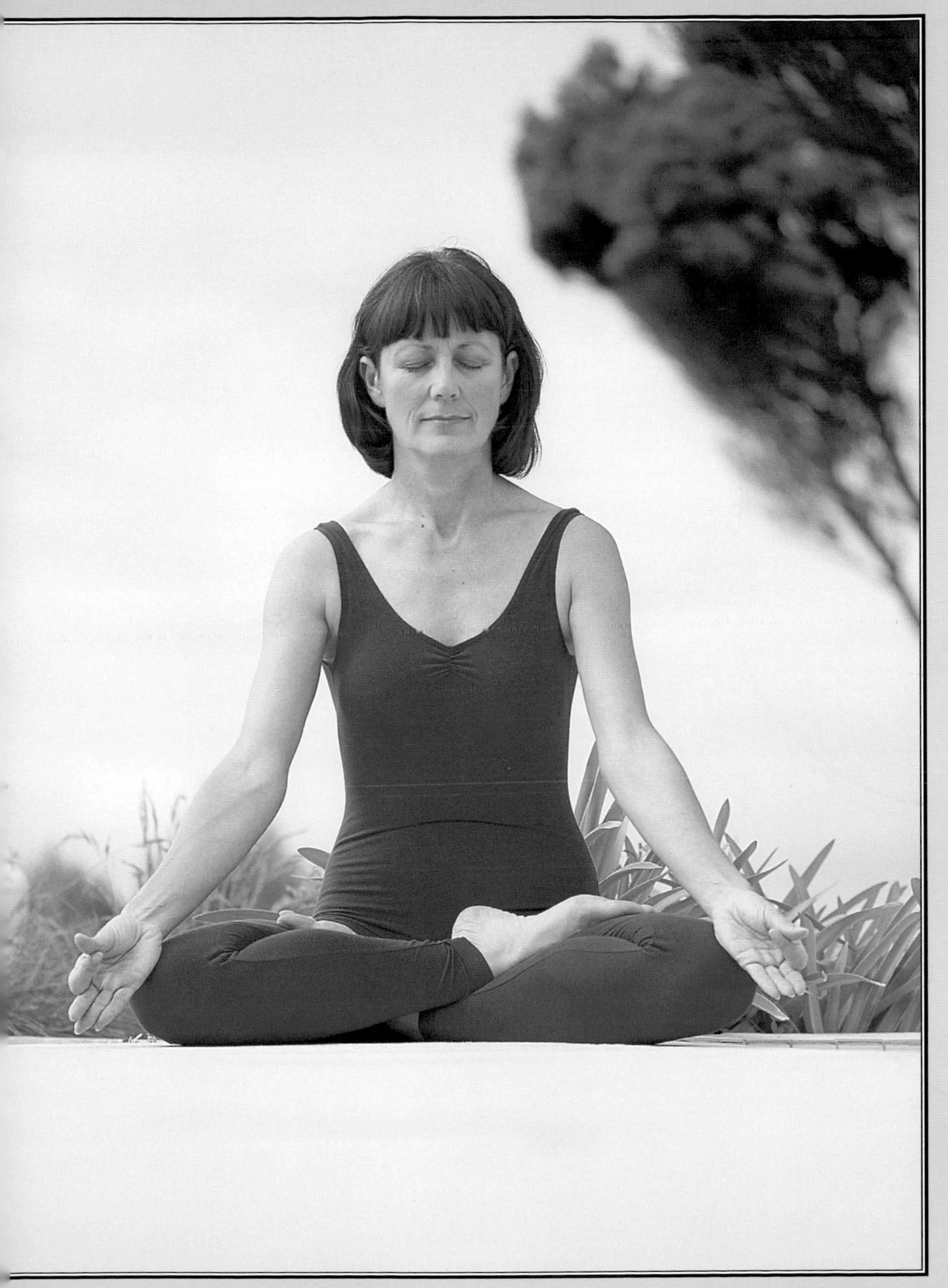

A Word on Diet

Just as daily practice of the physical postures promotes health and wellbeing, a sensible diet enables the body to obtain maximum benefit from the food you eat. Your body needs food to be able to repair itself, and as fuel for energy. Simple, natural and wholesome foods that are easily digested will enhance your journey toward radiant physical health.

Rather than making a sudden decision to change your eating habits, which might not be easy to maintain, simply listen more closely to your body's needs, and alter your diet gradually when you feel ready. A gentle approach to change is often more practical and sustainable than a hasty one. If you are in any doubt, consult your health practitioner for guidance as to the right food requirements for your particular metabolism.

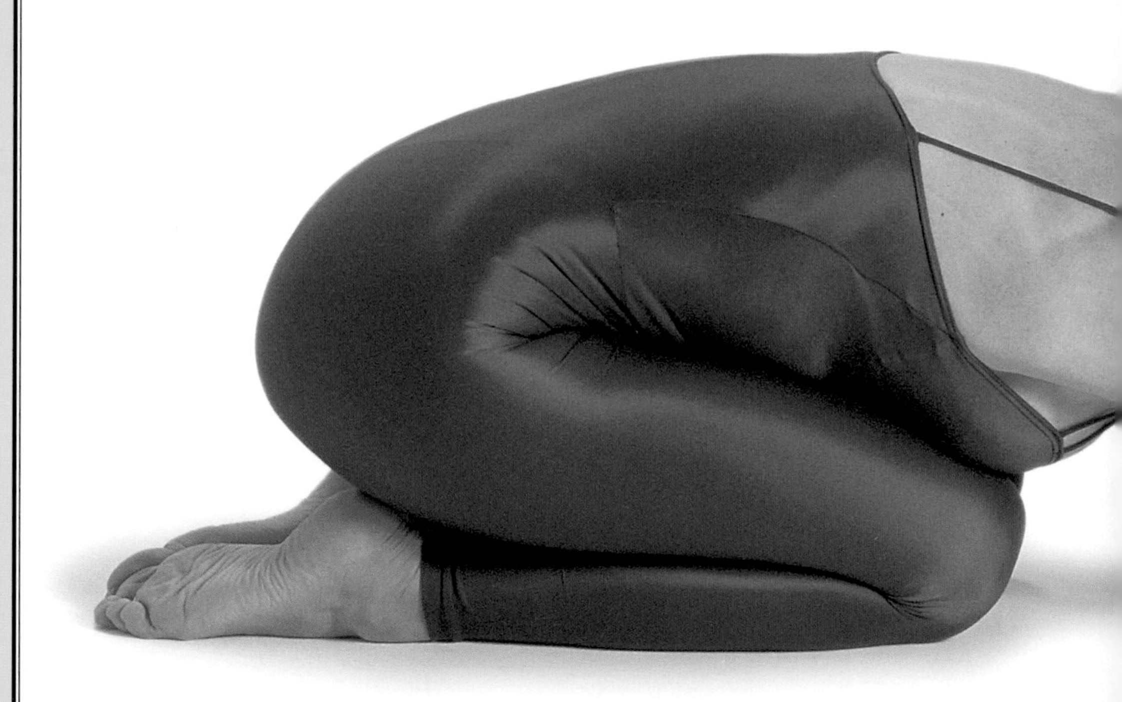

Conclusion

This book is a guide to yoga practice for those wishing to follow a routine at home. However there is no substitute for learning with a qualified yoga teacher. It is recommended that you take the time to find a teacher you can relate to and who teaches a style that is appropriate to your physical circumstances and also your temperament. You will discover that yoga teachers take many approaches. Some will focus more on the mental aspects, some on the devotional path, and others on the physical forms of yoga. The sequence we have described is based on a gentle physical style of Hatha yoga. Check in your local directory to see what yoga is available near you.

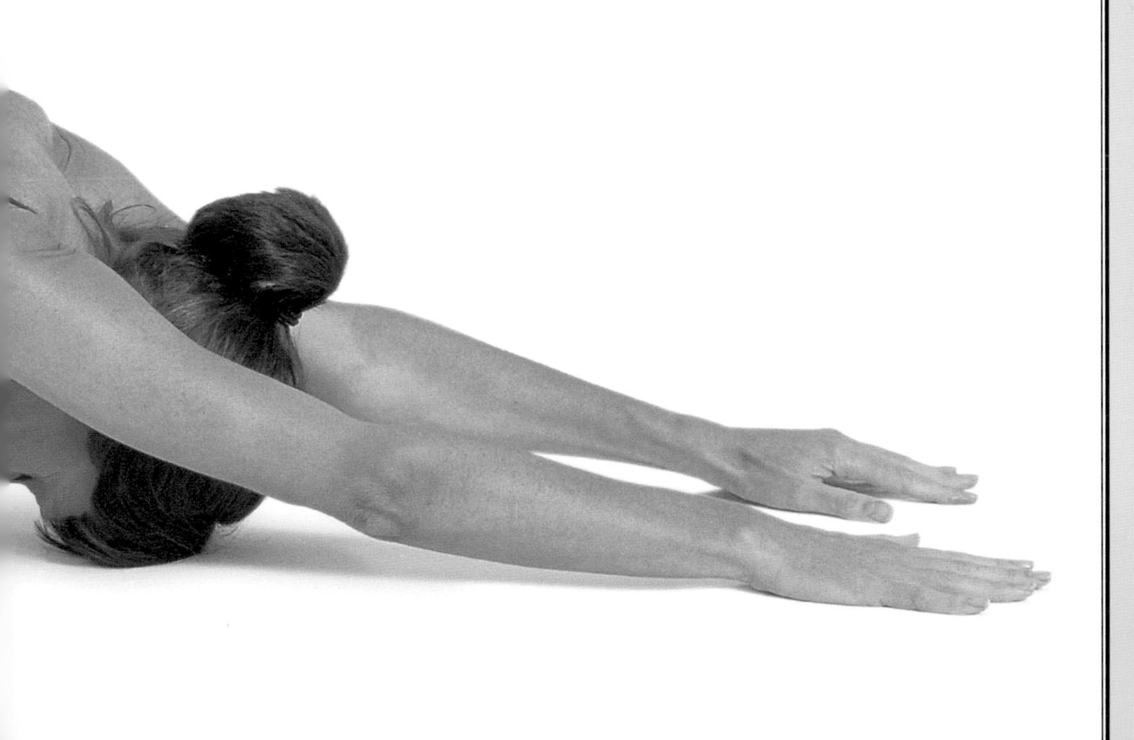

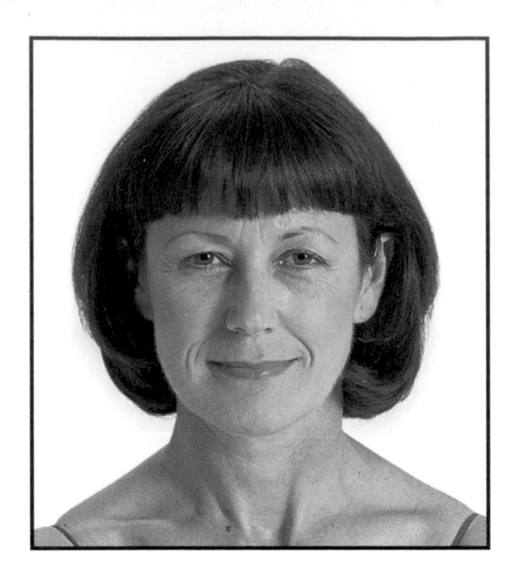

About the Author

When Yolanda Pettinato first discovered yoga she was in her mid-thirties. With no athletic or sporting background she could not even touch her toes. But she fell in love with yoga and took up formal studies both in Australia and in India. Now at 48, she teaches yoga from her studio in St Kilda, Melbourne. She hopes this book will encourage others to find good health, peace and harmony as she has, through yoga.